The
American Medical Association

GUIDE TO HEALTH AND WELL-BEING AFTER FIFTY

Revised and Updated Edition

The American Medical Association
Home Health Library

The American Medical Association
Family Medical Guide

The American Medical Association
Handbook of First Aid and Emergency Care

The American Medical Association
Guide to BackCare—Revised and Updated Edition

The American Medical Association
Guide to HeartCare—Revised and Updated Edition

The American Medical Association
Guide to WomanCare—Revised and Updated Edition

The American Medical Association
Guide to Health and Well-Being After Fifty

The American Medical Association
Guide to Better Sleep

The
American Medical Association

GUIDE TO
HEALTH AND
WELL-BEING
AFTER FIFTY

Revised and Updated Edition

Developed by the
American Medical Association

MEDICAL ADVISORS

Charles C. Edwards, M.D.

Roberta F. Fenlon, M.D.

Melvin Sabshin, M.D.

Written by Patricia Skalka

RANDOM HOUSE   NEW YORK

The recommendations and information in this book are appropriate in most cases. For specific information concerning your personal medical condition, however, the AMA suggests that you consult a physician. The names of organizations mentioned throughout this book are given for informational purposes only. Their inclusion implies neither approval nor disapproval by the AMA. To protect their privacy, the names of individuals cited in case studies have been changed.

Library of Congress Cataloging in Publication Data

Skalka, Patricia
The American Medical Association guide to health and
well-being after fifty

(American Medical Association home health library)
Includes bibliograhpical references and index.
1. Middle age—health and hygiene. I. American
Medical Association. II. Title. III. Title: Guide to
health and well-being after fifty. IV. Series. [DNLM:
1. Hygiene—In middle age—Popular works. 2. Middle age
—Popular works. WT 120 A512]
RA777.5.S58 1984   613'.0434   83-42759
ISBN 0-394-73829-2

Manufactured in the United States of America
24689753
First Edition

MEDICAL
ADVISORS

Charles C. Edwards, M.D., is president of the Scripps Clinic and Research Foundation, La Jolla, California. He is a former assistant secretary of the U.S. Department of Health, Education and Welfare (now the Department of Health and Human Services), and a former commissioner of the Food and Drug Administration. Dr. Edwards, a native of Kearney, Nebraska, received his M.D. from the University of Colorado School of Medicine, Boulder. He is a Fellow of the American College of Surgeons and a diplomate of the American Board of Surgery.

Roberta F. Fenlon, M.D., is an internist in private practice in San Francisco, California, and is clinical professor of medicine at the University of California. She is a past president of the California Medical Association and a former editor of the Association's medical journal. Born in Clinton, Iowa, Dr. Fenlon received her M.D. from the University of Iowa College of Medicine, Iowa City. She is a member of several national professional associations, including the American Society of Internal Medicine and the American College of Physicians.

Melvin Sabshin, M.D., is medical director of the American Psychiatric Association, Washington, D.C. He is a former professor and head of the department of psychiatry at the University of Illinois College of Medicine, Urbana, and a past president of the

American College of Psychiatrists. A native of New York City, Dr. Sabshin received his M.D. from Tulane University, New Orleans, Louisiana. He is a member of several medical specialty societies, including the Group for the Advancement of Psychiatry and the American Psychosomatic Society.

American Medical Association Consumer Book Program
Thomas F. Hannon, Deputy Executive Vice President, AMA
John T. Baker, Vice President, Publishing, AMA
Charles C. Renshaw, Jr., Editorial Director, Consumer Book Program, AMA

PREFACE

Surely the most valuable asset we Americans have, both as individuals and as a nation, is our health. Good health is the cornerstone of almost every productive human activity. Yet all too often we squander our health, either by neglecting our physical and emotional needs or by indulging in habits that are patently harmful.

In recent decades our failure to adequately maintain our health has been largely obscured by the fanfare surrounding the introduction of a host of new "wonder drugs" and an imposing array of advanced medical technology. But these innovations, despite the many benefits they have brought us, are not adequate by themselves to meet our health needs and aspirations. Something more is required, something important.

It is now clear beyond doubt that if we wish to enjoy the attributes of continued good health in the years ahead, the impetus will have to come from each of us, working as individuals in our own best interests. As individuals, each of us is better qualified than anyone else to act as the guardian of his or her health. By looking within ourselves and adopting prudent health habits and sensible life-styles, we can prevent unnecessary illness, needless loss of vitality and premature old age or death.

There is, moreover, an economic urgency about all this, an urgency that affects every one of us. For a variety of reasons, medical costs have risen to unprecedented levels. Certainly one of the most effective ways the individual can help to combat this problem is to avoid what is avoidable and to prevent what is preventable.

These are the reasons that have motivated the American Medical Association, in collaboration with Random House, to publish this book. It is one of a series of books, collectively entitled *The American Medical Association Home Health Library*, which bring you the latest, most authoritative and useful information on a wide range of health-care subjects. As doctors, we firmly believe that if you are given the facts, and the professional guidance necessary to understand and apply those facts, you will act wisely in your own behalf.

There are approximately 23 million men and women in the United States in the fifties age group, a number that represents over 10 percent of our total population. If you are among this group, there is much you can do not only to prevent unnecessary illness but also to enhance your enjoyment of life. Regardless of age, it is never too late to adopt a sensible, healthful way of life.

We at the AMA look upon this book as an important opportunity to talk directly with those of you who are in your fifties about your health. We believe that once you are equipped with sound and balanced information, you will be able to shape a better, more fruitful life for yourself and those closest to you. That is certainly our hope.

James H. Sammons, M.D.
Executive Vice President
American Medical Association

ACKNOWLEDGMENTS

The publication of *The American Medical Association Guide to Health and Well-Being After Fifty* would not have been possible without the cooperation and generous help of the many men and women who contributed their time and expertise to the book's development.

We owe special gratitude to Drs. Charles C. Edwards, Roberta F. Fenlon and Melvin Sabshin, who helped guide the book from its inception and whose scientific knowledge and dedication to excellence have been invaluable.

We also wish to thank the many physicians and health professionals quoted throughout the text for their expert information, and we particularly want to acknowledge the valuable assistance provided by the following individuals and institutions: William L. Beery (Chapel Hill, North Carolina); Ann Dugan (Evanston, Illinois); Douglas Gasner (Chicago, Illinois); Robin B. Goldsmith (La Jolla, California); Clyde C. Greene, Jr., M.D. (San Francisco, California); D. R. Inge (San Francisco, California); the late Vernon Inman, M.D. (Santa Clara, California); Edward A. Krull, M.D. (Detroit, Michigan); Deborah Szekely Mazzanti (San Diego, California); Kathleen Peterson (Chicago, Illinois); Elizabeth A. Regan, R.N. (Oshkosh, Wisconsin); Dan Rogers (Baltimore, Maryland); Sally Rynne (Evanston, Illinois); Gary D. Scherer (La Jolla, California); H. Scott Sheedy (Indianapolis, Indiana); Richard E. Stiefler, M.D. (Detroit, Michigan); the late Jack Weinberg,

M.D. (Chicago, Illinois); and the late Leon Zussman, M.D. (New York, New York). Also the American Association of Retired Persons; The Clearing, operated by the Wisconsin Farm Bureau Federation (Ellison Bay, Wisconsin); the Forty Plus Club of Chicago (Chicago, Illinois); Rancho la Puerto (Tecate, Mexico); and the National Institute on Aging.

And, to Charles A. Wimpfheimer, Klara Glowczewski and Bernard Klein of Random House, our gratitude for their knowledgeable guidance and support.

We also wish to express our gratitude to the following members of the AMA's editorial team for their creativity, skill and insistence on high quality: Patricia Skalka, Kathleen A. Kaye, Robin Fitzpatrick, Ralph L. Linnenburger, David LaHoda, Sophie Klim, Virginia J. Peterson and Marie Moore.

In addition, we want to thank the men and women who graciously shared their mid-life experiences with us and with the readers of this book. Their contribution has been significant, and we are very grateful to them.

Carole A. Fina
Managing Editor
American Medical Association
Consumer Book Program

CONTENTS

LIST OF
ILLUSTRATIONS

INTRODUCTION

WHY A HEALTH CARE BOOK ON THE FIFTIES?

Not too long ago, when astronaut John Young successfully commanded the first U.S. space shuttle, he was fifty years old. In that historic undertaking, Young scored a victory not only for his country but also for middle-aged men and women. The pilot of the *Columbia* showed the world an image of a fifty-year-old that was at direct odds with the common stereotype. Along with other newsmakers and celebrities of his age group, astronaut Young helped focus public attention on an exciting and vital decade of life that medical experts and social scientists agree has been the most often ignored and misunderstood.

At the turn of the century when people traveled by horseback and steam-powered train, the average life expectancy in this country was forty-nine years of age. Now, fifty-year-olds sit at the controls of four-million-ton space vehicles. How did this incredible metamorphosis come about?

There is no one simple answer to the question. Many factors were involved. Advancements in health care, improvements in working conditions and upswings in educational and socioeconomic standards have all contributed to the tremendous extension of life expectancy and to the social developments that have occurred during the last three quarters of a century.

The fifties decade has been transformed from old age to middle age, from a passive to an active period of life. Today's fifty-year-olds are on the cutting edge of change. More options are open to them in every avenue of human endeavor. They have more public resources at their disposal than past generations would have dreamed possible. And they have more personal freedom and more years of living to anticipate, plan for and enjoy than any preceding generation.

Numbers alone distinguish the current group of fifty-year-olds. There are 23 million Americans in the fifties age bracket. That figure is equal to the combined populations of the entire metropolitan areas of New York City, Los Angeles and Chicago. Today's fifty-year-olds represent approximately 10 percent of the country's total population, a fact that enables them, for example, to influence both local and national elections. Economically, they and their older colleagues control more than half the discretionary income in this country and in Canada.

In terms of health, the new breed of middle-aged men and women is also unique. They are the beneficiaries of a knowledge explosion in the field of medicine that has significantly contributed to a better understanding of the aging process and to more effective prevention and treatment of human disease. They are in a position to have a positive impact on their overall well-being. According to a report from the U.S. Surgeon General, individuals today can greatly influence many adult health problems, often through relatively simple measures.

In general, we are experiencing a shift from an overall negative to a generally positive view of middle age. This attitude shift results in large part from an important change in the focus of medical research. Traditionally, knowledge about the aging process was gathered from studies and case histories of relatively small groups of people, usually medical patients. Today, many theories of aging are based on long-range studies of subjects who are normal, healthy individuals or on surveys of large samples of people drawn from cross sections of the general public.

Medicine's view of the aging process has changed dramatically. As the picture of "normal aging" comes more clearly into focus, misconceptions and dreary generalizations are discarded. For today's fifty-year-olds, a new optimism prevails.

Human-development expert Bernice L. Neugarten, Ph.D., of Northwestern University, Chicago, Illinois, voices the scientific community's new, more positive attitude toward mid-life.

• First, she says, it does not do justice to men and women to describe middle age only in terms of problems and not also in terms of freedoms and gains.

• Second, most people who have reached middle age do not wish to be young again, even though they may wish to feel young. Men and women in middle age want instead to grow old with equanimity and with the assurance that they will have a full measure of life's experiences.

Traditionally, society functioned under the assumption that life became increasingly empty and less meaningful as one approached middle age. Not so, says Dr. Neugarten, "With the passage of time, life becomes more, not less, complex. It becomes enriched, not impoverished."

"I realize with astonishment that this is the happiest time of my life," writes Sloan Wilson, author of *The Man in the Grey Flannel Suit*. In fact, says Wilson, who is sixty, his own life did not start "to get better" until he reached age fifty.

"I know that everyone is supposed to think that youth is marvelous," he says, "but, when I try to remember the past accurately, I realize that I had a cold much of the time when I was in my teens, suffered the usual skin problems and was convinced that I was stupid and ugly." Young adulthood brought a world war that, despite all the comedies written about it, says Wilson, "was not really all that much fun." After the war came the task of earning a living, a challenge that, in his words, "sometimes seemed even harder than the other battles."

Now, finally, says Wilson, he feels he is smart, sassy looking and happy. "The idea that life must necessarily get worse and worse after age thirty or forty or fifty presupposes that experience means nothing and that accumulated knowledge is useless." That, he notes, is true only for people who can't learn.

Indeed, many men and women agree that they view middle age as a fulfilling time. A study headed by John C. Flanagan, Ph.D., founder of the American Institutes for Research, an independent educational and health research organization in Palo Alto, California, found that, of 800 fifty-year-old men and women asked to rate their overall quality of life as "poor," "fair," "good," "very good" or "excellent," nearly 87 percent chose the designations "good," "very good" or "excellent." In two decades of research at the

University of Michigan Institute for Social Research, Ann Arbor, investigators have found that "one of the most satisfying times of life is the later period—ages forty-five and up—when children have grown up and left home and the parents are still married and living together." And, at the Center for the Study of Aging and Human Development at Duke University Medical Center, Durham, North Carolina, an analysis of life satisfaction shows that, contrary to existing theory, mid-life is a period of "overall stability."

Peter V. Sacks, M.D., head of the Division of Preventive Medicine at Scripps Clinic and Research Foundation, La Jolla, California, offers the following words of advice for men and women who have reached middle age:

> You have a right to your high expectations about the quality of life you enjoy during the middle years. But you have to work toward this goal. By accepting personal responsibility for your life-style and health habits, and, consequently, for your own well-being, you help ensure that you will enjoy the best return and the highest level of satisfaction from your fifties.

In the pages that follow, we will address the question of how you in the fifties age group can best utilize your individual physiological and psychological resources to enjoy a satisfying, comfortable middle age and avoid premature old age. To bring you the most reliable and up-to-date advice, we have interviewed physicians, mental health professionals, aging and development researchers and a host of experts whose various fields of endeavor are concerned with issues of the mid-life period.

According to their findings, the depth and richness of our lives as we enter and move through middle age are influenced by specific, identifiable traits: good health, an ability to cope with limitations, flexible attitudes, personal resources, well-being and a sense of future.

• *Good health.* There is much that you as an individual can do to remain healthy and vital throughout both your middle and your later years. Physicians recommend several steps:

  1. Have regular, routine medical checkups.
  2. Adhere to a program of sensible exercise and eating habits.

3. Remain mentally active and avoid major risk factors (these are discussed in Chapter 1).

4. Comply with your physician's directions for treatment.

• *An ability to cope with limitations.* Few of us will enter our fifties without experiencing some decline or alteration in physical function. If you acknowledge and accept your own physiological limitations, you can learn how to compensate for diminished talents and how to make the most of your existing capabilities. The result can be a healthful, active and more satisfying period of life.

• *Flexible attitudes.* In later chapters we discuss some of the changes in personal circumstances and values that can generate a need for new activities, goals and interests in mid-life. Transitions and life-altering events are inescapable. If you are to thrive, you must learn to bend. You must develop a flexible attitude toward life and recognize that more elements than you may realize come under your personal control and influence. Despite misconceptions to the contrary, people *can* change.

• *Personal resources.* A flexible attitude provides the key to change, but personal resources furnish the means for self-renewal and growth. At mid-life, shifting gears and beginning to restructure your life-style may seem an overwhelming task, but such is often not the case. In fact, you rarely have to look far for the means to self-renewal. Each of us has a variety of talents and interests long forgotten or ignored, and rediscovering your own potentials will add new depth and dimension to the middle years and will enrich the quality of your life.

• *Well-being.* Swiss physician and psychologist Dr. Paul Tournier associates well-being with the feeling of fulfillment you experience when you accomplish a task, when you have a goal and the hope of achieving that goal. Well-being arises when you function at optimum physical and mental capacity and when you make the most of your opportunities and potential.

• *A sense of future.* Throughout your life, you need a sense of purpose. When you are younger, your roles are usually prescribed by society—to be a parent, an entrepreneur, a worker. But, by mid-life, you have often fulfilled these roles, and the larger question arises: Now what? If you are to find happiness and fulfillment and maintain self-esteem, you must develop new roles that will give meaning to your life. In doing so, you create what Judith

Bardwick, Ph.D., of the University of Michigan, Ann Arbor, labels "a sense of future."

At mid-life, says Dr. Bardwick, a professor of psychology, your sense of future is tied directly to the personal commitments you make, both to yourself and to society. "It seems necessary to believe that it will be a good, moral thing for you to achieve. It seems necessary to initiate and control change, for then change for its own sake is perceived as exhilarating. It seems necessary to experience yourself as coping and as becoming." If we achieve these ends, we then embrace middle age with maturity and strength.

To live to the fullest during the fifties decade, you will need accurate information about both your physical and your psychological capabilities. Misconceptions, myths and half-truths not only distort reality, they also generate fears that inhibit actions and limit dreams.

You will need faith in yourself, and this comes from knowledge of yourself: from self-awareness, from being responsive to change and from having a sense of the future. You also need mentors and the inspiration their experiences provide.

Robert J. Havinghurst, Ph.D., professor emeritus at the University of Chicago and a pioneer in aging research, calls the fifties the most critical and challenging decade of life. Throughout this book, you will see why and how it can also be one of the richest and most rewarding.

The
American Medical Association

GUIDE TO
HEALTH AND
WELL-BEING
AFTER FIFTY

Revised and Updated Edition

1

GOOD NEWS ABOUT HEALTH AND VITALITY IN MID-LIFE

Some of the most sophisticated research on aging is being conducted in a four-story brick building that looks more like a twentieth-century version of the little red schoolhouse than a modern scientific laboratory. The facility is the Gerontology Research Center of the National Institute on Aging, Baltimore, Maryland. Funded by $16 million annually from the National Institutes of Health, some 175 permanent staff members devote their energies and expertise to unraveling and understanding just what it means to grow old. They are still far from solving all the mysteries, but they have accumulated more knowledge on aging than ever before. Some of what they have learned is surprising, most of it is reassuring and all of it will one day benefit the human race in ways we can now only speculate about.

At one end of the research complex, the researchers study laboratory animals; at the other end, humans. It is here, following an elaborately prepared schedule, that 650 men and 150 women, ranging in age from their early twenties to mid-nineties, report regularly for three days of examinations and tests. They walk treadmills, breathe into special monitoring devices and squeeze handgrips to demonstrate how much, if at all, their physical performance alters over time. Some are injected with glucose solutions, others with a pure alcohol solution to determine tolerance levels. They are monitored by a cadre of machines that measure virtually every body part, from the heart to the tiny blood vessels in the retina. They undergo both physical and mental tests, and many will volunteer to come back again and repeat the process at twelve-, eighteen- or twenty-four-month intervals.

The work in progress at the Baltimore center and at other gerontological research facilities is really a modern version of an ancient quest, an attempt to answer a question that has been asked for centuries: Why do we age?

To date, no one knows for sure. There are a number of theories, of course. It is possible, for example, that somewhere in the brain a master mechanism determines and directs the aging process through its control over the body's hormonal system. It is possible, too, that aging's clock lies in individual cells and is linked to genetic coding. Another theory, falling out of favor today, blames lipofuscin, or fatty-pigment accumulation, a kind of self-pollution. And then there is the principle of wear and tear, which dictates that unless a part is replaced or repaired, it will one day fail.

All of these factors—and more—play a part in aging. The difficulty comes in assigning proper importance to each and determining a correct sequence of events. Eventually, we will know enough to be able to combat or deter the changes we wish to avoid. Today we are still trying to understand the process. In the meantime, scientists are uncovering interesting findings and debunking a few myths along the way.

According to Nathan W. Shock, Ph.D., founder and former chief of the Gerontology Research Center, there are two popular notions about aging that scientists now know are not true:

• First, aging is not a phenomenon that suddenly descends upon us during the middle years. Unless accelerated by disease, the aging process progresses gradually over time. In other words, you probably have "aged" as much in the past twenty years as you will in the next two decades. Since you have been growing old right along, aging is not a new experience to which you must adapt immediately at this point in your life. You have, in fact, been adapting for a lifetime. The big difference is that, as the years pass, you accumulate more changes, so the total impact may seem greater by mid-life.

• Second, aging does not cause illness. Until recently, aging and illness were considered almost synonymous. You grow old; you become sick. But this is not true. *Normal* aging does not by definition include the development of disease. In other words, if you age normally, you will grow older while remaining healthy. True, many elderly persons become ill, but their illnesses are in many cases not caused by advanced age. Invariably other culprits can be identified.

What aging in and of itself brings about are demonstrable changes in appearance and a decline in bodily functions. No part of the body escapes the aging process. Some of the alterations are external and highly visible: hair turns gray, skin sags, wrinkles set in. Others are internal. We become aware of them indirectly when we notice a difference in the way we act or feel. At the Baltimore center, scientists work to quantify the changes we can't see. They have found that complex functions of the body, such as using arm and shoulder muscles to turn a crank in smooth, coordinated fashion, are affected more adversely by age than are the simple processes, such as using those same muscles to push or pull a stationary object. Research also shows that each bodily system responds differently to aging. For example:

The Cardiovascular System	The amount of blood pumped by the heart decreases with age. Assuming the heart functions at 100 percent capacity at age thirty, its efficiency is down to 80 percent by age fifty and 70 percent by age eighty. Blood pressure tends to rise, and resting heart rate declines. Structurally, the heart loses some muscle fibers, while insoluble granular material (proteins and lipids, or fats) tends to accumulate. Blood vessels also thicken and become less elastic. Arteriosclerosis, or hardening of the arteries, generally occurs to some extent by mid-life.
The Pulmonary System	Breathing capacity by age fifty is down to 75 percent (compared with 100 percent at age thirty), and

useful lung volume has dropped to 80 percent. Structurally the lungs lose some of their elasticity with age. In addition, the bony chest cage becomes stiffer and the muscles that move the chest during inhalation and exhalation tend to become weaker.

The Nervous System

The speed at which a nerve impulse travels from the brain to a muscle fiber somewhere in the body decreases only by about 10 percent over the course of an entire lifetime. By age fifty, it has slowed to half that figure, or a mere 5 percent. Structural changes in the brain at this point are negligible. For the average individual, noticeable changes usually affect the sensory organs, most noticeably the eyes and ears, but rarely to an extent that cannot be corrected with glasses and hearing aids.

To the uninitiated, the changes may seem extensive. To the researchers at the Gerontology Research Center, the results represent a surprisingly minimal amount of change. Even more encouraging are the facts that:

• All the figures are averages. This means that the amount of decline experienced by an individual man or woman may be much less than the average.

• The rate of change varies tremendously from one person to another. For example, some seventy-year-old people tested at the Baltimore facility had the reactions of individuals twenty years younger.

Ultimately, you will become aware that it takes you more time to adapt to physiological stress and exertion. With exercise, for example, heart rate, blood pressure, respiration and oxygen consumption are increased, whether you are age thirty or fifty-five. But if you are thirty, chances are that your body returns to its normal rate of function after two or three minutes. If you are fifty-five, you will need more time to recover from the same amount of activity.

If you are in good health, there is no reason you should curtail or drastically alter your physical activities just because you have reached middle age, says Dr. Shock, who was born in 1906. But research findings indicate that, for the sake of your physical well-being and to avoid pushing your body to a point of maximum stress, you should alter your approach to physical exertion. For instance, you should

• Accept the fact that level of functioning has changed. There is a hazard for the fifty-year-old man who says, "Oh hell, I'm just as good as I ever was." He isn't.

• Give yourself more time in which to complete and recuperate from physical activity. For example, allow a rest period between a lunch-hour workout and your return to the office. Sit and relax for fifteen or twenty minutes between tennis matches. Schedule quiet time between vigorous housecleaning and lawn work.

As research data accumulate, scientists continue to learn more about the normal process of human aging. They know, for example, that in late life it is not unusual for the body's immune and auditory systems to be slightly impaired. That is why the elderly are more susceptible to disease and loss of hearing. They know that, by middle age, the body's enzyme and hormone detector systems become less sensitive. For years scientists thought that age slowly rendered the systems inoperative. They now know this is not true: The mechanisms generally function well, but by mid-life it takes more of a stimulus to trigger the proper reaction. Thus, sexual response time increases. So, too, does the amount of time required for blood sugar levels to return to normal after sugar is ingested.

These types of research findings are important, because for the first time researchers know that the criteria for determining "normal function" change over time. They understand that it is misleading to compare a fifty-year-old with a thirty-year-old and that standards of normal good health should vary from one age group to another.

For the middle-aged, this is encouraging news. It means you are judged by standards appropriate for your age and not for any other. It means you can be healthy at age fifty-five even if you do not demonstrate the same reactions and function levels as someone a decade younger.

What about aging and the mind? Is it true, for example, as scientific and lay mythology once professed, that we reach an intellectual peak at about age thirty, maintain the plateau for a few years, then start on a downward trend, bottoming out in our sixties? Not according to the findings of the Baltimore researchers.

The researchers have learned that, while some decline occurs in memory, learning and reasoning, it happens only late in life—usually after age seventy—and again with wide differences in individuals. "We don't know if everyone experiences such a decline mentally," says David Arenberg, Ph.D., chief of the learning and problem-solving section at the Gerontology Research Center's Laboratory of Behavioral Sciences. "We have seen individuals who have not during the six or twelve years they've been studied." He also cautions that the types of changes he and his colleagues look at involve performance alterations in laboratory tasks, not the things you'd notice in conversation. "It may be," he admits, "that the kind of things we pick up really aren't that important in terms of day-to-day functioning."

According to a theory developed in the 1960s by psychologists Raymond B. Cattell, Ph.D., of the University of Hawaii, Honolulu, and John L. Horn, Ph.D., of the University of Denver, human beings have two kinds of intelligence. The first they term *fluid intelligence.* It deals with new information. The other is *crystallized intelligence.* This kind is concerned with old information—the accumulated knowledge from past experience.

According to research at the Baltimore center, age seems to have no effect on activities that depend on old information. However, age does tend to affect the way we deal with new information, whether we are trying to learn, remember or reason with it. Says Dr. Arenberg, it may be more difficult to acquire new information as you get older, but that doesn't mean you can't learn. What you may need more of are motivation—is it worth it to you to make the effort to acquire this particular knowledge?—and time, since the process may take you longer than in earlier years.

Good physical health and activity both appear instrumental in preserving mental acuity. Although there is no scientific proof that supports the latter's role in maintaining intellectual sparkle, the theory is embraced by scientists both in this country and in others. In test animals, research at Jackson Laboratory (a private research facility devoted primarily to mammalian genetics research) in Bar Harbor, Maine, shows that physical condition, not age, is the determining factor of both intelligence quotient (IQ) and learning ability. Whether this is true or not for humans remains to be proved, but tests are already under way.

In a preliminary analysis at the Gerontology Research Center, memory and blood pressure were studied to determine if hypertension has a deleterious effect on cognitive performance. (According to one theory, high blood pressure could negatively affect oxygenation of the brain and thus impair functioning.) In the future, as more data are accrued, scientists expect to have more definitive answers about possible cause-and-effect relationships between general health and cognitive performance.

What we need not fear is that our brains will deteriorate seriously as we age. Brain cells do die—at the amazing rate of some 50,000 cells per day—but the amount is insignificant compared with the number of cells in the brain. Furthermore, the brain is composed of many different types of cells. Only certain types die, and, because of natural interaction, others compensate for the lost cells and take over their functions. In the absence of diseases that directly affect neuron functions in the brain, we are basically assured that our minds, like our bodies, can age gracefully.

In the final analysis, there is, of course, nothing to be gained by stating that decrements and impairments do not occur with age, because they do. But in the absence of disease the changes take place gradually and allow us time to develop many adaptive measures. In terms of performance we can, in effect, avoid the primary effects of age-related changes. But we must strive for this goal. "The way you react and respond to any impairment, no matter how slight, will have a great effect on your life," says Dr. Shock. "The worst thing you can do is nurse the impairment and let it become a major influence in your life. The best thing you can do is accept it as part of your life-style and put up with it. You are always better off maintaining physical and mental activity, even in the face of some inconvenience or discomfort."

Growing Older While Remaining Healthy

If at age fifty you are going to have an impact on how aging affects you, it will be in the realm of prevention. This is because most of the physiological changes you experience as you grow older, while not reversible, can often be prevented or postponed.

For example, according to the National Center for Health Statistics, in 1970 the death rate in the United States for adults aged twenty-five to sixty-four was 657 per 100,000. By 1977, the rate had dropped to 540 per 100,000, primarily because of a decline in heart attacks and strokes, attributed largely to the detection and control of high blood pressure, reduction in smoking, increase in exercise and other life-style changes.

One of the first large-scale studies to demonstrate the value of controlling high blood pressure was conducted by the Veterans Administration Cooperative Study Group. In one phase of the project, 380 hypertensive men were monitored for five years. Of those who controlled their elevated blood pressure levels, only 19 percent experienced any cardiovascular disturbance. Among the men whose hypertension was not controlled, 55 percent developed heart disease. More recently, 10,940 hypertensive adults, aged thirty to sixty-nine, participated in the nationwide Hypertension Detection and Follow-up Program sponsored by the National Institutes of Health. Again, among the participants who successfully lowered blood pressure levels by following prescribed antihypertensive therapies, death rates after five years were significantly lowered.

You can have a similar impact on lessening your chances of developing lung cancer. Let us assume that you are a fifty-year-old man who decides to quit smoking. You toss out the pack, wash the ashtrays and never take another puff on a cigarette. You have no guarantee of avoiding the number-one cancer killer for men in the country—lung cancer—but by approximately age fifty-seven you will have reduced by one-half your chances of getting the disease. By the time you are sixty-five years old, you will have brought down the odds to less than 1 percent, the same as those for a man who has never smoked. There's even an added bonus, according to researchers at the Gerontology Research Center. As a fifty-year-old smoker, you had the lung function of a man ten to fifteen years older. But within one or two years of quitting smoking, your lung capacity will equal that of the average nonsmoker your age. (It should be noted, however, that in some cases damage to the alveoli—the air cells of the lungs—is irreversible.)

Even when exact preventive techniques are still unknown, there is hope in early detection and treatment. A case in point is breast cancer. Consider the facts:

- Breast cancer is the major cancer killer of women in this country. (Although men are also victims of breast cancer, less than 5 percent of the instances of the disease occurs in males.)
- Its main target is the woman—and man—over age thirty-five.
- Breast cancer survival rates can be directly proportional to how early treatment is sought.

Cancer cells vary; some are more aggressive than others, complicating prognosis and subsequent treatment. In a National Cancer Institute study of 2,039 women whose cancers shared certain characteristics, however, tumor size was related to survival. According to the findings, 80 percent of the women who were treated for breast cancer tumors that were less than 1 centimeter in diameter were alive ten years later. Only 55 percent of those with tumors of 3 to 4 centimeters, and 45 percent with tumors of 5 to 7½ centimeters, survived for the same length of time. (It should be noted, however, that, while early detection of cancer is critical, the *biological nature* of the cancer at any stage plays an extremely important role.)

Data from the American Cancer Society indicate that women themselves can be their own best defense against the disease. According to the society, approximately 95 percent of all breast cancers are first detected by women, often through use of the breast self-examination (see the next page for details).

"The problem with most of us is that we don't want to think about our bodies, because to consider the body means to consider its mortality," says Ernest L. Wynder, M.D., president of the American Health Foundation, New York. "This is one of the mental obstacles to preventive medicine."

If we realize, however, that we can take action to prolong our

Breast Self-Examination

The following five-step procedure is recommended by the National Cancer Institute.

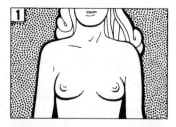

1. Stand before a mirror and inspect both breasts for anything unusual, such as any discharge from the nipples, puckering, dimpling or scaling of the skin.

2. The next two steps are designed to emphasize any change in the shape or contour of your breast. As you do them, you should be able to feel your chest muscles tighten. Watching closely in the mirror, clasp hands behind your head and press hands forward.

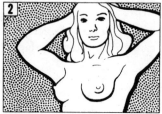

3. Next, press hands firmly on hips and bow slightly toward your mirror as you pull your shoulders and elbows forward.

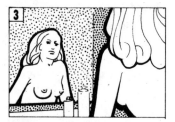

4. Some women do the next part of the exam in the shower. Fingers glide over soapy skin, making it easy to concentrate on the texture underneath.

   Raise your left arm. Use three or four fingers of your right hand to firmly, and carefully explore your left breast. Beginning at the outer edge, press your fingers in small circles, moving the circles slowly around the breast. Gradually work toward the nipple. Be sure to cover the entire breast. Pay special attention to the area between the breast and the armpit, including the armpit itself. Feel for any unusual lump or mass under the skin. Gently squeeze the nipple and look for a discharge. Repeat the exam on your right breast.

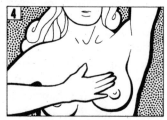

5. If you wish to perform the exam lying down, lie flat on your back with your left arm over your head and a pillow or folded towel under your left shoulder. This flattens the breast and makes it easier to examine. Use the same circular motion described earlier. Repeat the exam on your right breast. You might want to try both positions—standing or lying down—to see which is more comfortable for you. The most important choice is the decision to do the breast self-examination each month.

   If you menstruate, the best time to perform the exam is at the end of your period, when your breasts are least likely to be tender or swollen. If you are menopausal or postmenopausal, you may find it helpful to pick a day, such as the first day of the month.

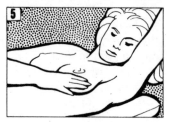

lives, then our attitude might change. Imagine dying young—of old age! That is what nature intended, and the earlier in life we conduct ourselves properly the better chance we have of attaining that end. "For the middle-aged person, the number-one interest should be improving his or her life-style to prevent diseases from getting into full bloom." To ensure continued good health, you should take the following steps:

• Have regular checkups. These should include checks for blood-lipid levels and blood pressure, and Pap smears for women. How often you should have these examinations depends largely on how much your results deviate from the norm. This will be determined by your physician. When asked about personal life-style habits, give honest appraisals about the extent of smoking and drinking you engage in and how much you exercise.

• Develop a personalized health history. This should include the health histories of your parents and other relatives as well as your medical history, any hospitalizations or surgical procedures and a list of the medications you take. The information can be helpful to a physician treating you for medical problems that may arise at a later date. (See the Appendix: Your Personal Health History.)

• Become familiar with major disease risk factors and determine what steps you can take to avoid those factors that can reasonably be avoided. For example, the key risk factors for coronary heart disease are blood-lipid levels, high blood pressure and smoking. The lower these values are and the less you smoke, the less risk you have of developing a heart attack.

In a landmark study headed by Lester Breslow, M.D., dean of the School of Public Health at the University of California, Los Angeles, the health status and life-style habits of 6,928 adults in Alameda County, California, were analyzed to determine what identifiable factors contributed to the participants' health and, in turn, what detracted from their physical well-being. Altogether, researchers isolated seven basic practices that can enhance a person's health at any given time and that are directly associated with one's life expectancy. The health practices are:

1. Don't smoke cigarettes.
2. If you drink, do it moderately.
3. Eat breakfast.
4. Don't eat between meals.

5. Maintain normal weight.
6. Sleep about eight hours each night.
7. Exercise moderately.

The health habits are not news in and of themselves. However, the California study has quantified, for the first time, the potential impact of adhering to these rules. According to Dr. Breslow's initial reports: "At any age—from age twenty up to seventy-five years—the health of people with seven good health habits was better than that of people with six. Health of the latter was better than that of those with only five and so on, consistently with four, three and two or fewer good health habits." This was true no matter what the occupation, income level or sex of the subjects.

For the middle-aged, findings from the California study translate into good, solid health news. If you are fifty-five to sixty-four years old and follow the seven basic practices, then physically your health status might equal that of someone twenty-five to thirty-four years old. If you are a woman and maintain this life-style, you can add as much as seven years to your life span. If you are a man and adhere to the principles, you can add eleven to twelve years to your life. The more you cheat, the more you lose. The harder you try, the more you gain.

2

NEW WAYS TO REDUCE RISKS OF SICKNESS AND DISEASE

Bonnie Simmons is a walking contradiction. She is simultaneously fifty-three and forty-eight years old, and she is in a position to possibly—and rather remarkably—grow younger. In fact, Bonnie has been told that, if she makes a few changes in her life-style, she can lower her age to forty-six. Bonnie is not the victim of some quick, gimmick-promoting huckster. The information she has been given is based on scientific fact and represents one of the great breakthroughs in modern medicine.

Bonnie Simmons has before her a personalized health analysis. The analysis takes into account factors about her life-style, family history and health data and combines these with the known risks for people her age, race and sex. It produces a profile that gives Bonnie her current and potential health status and tells her how she can improve both.

Chronologically, Bonnie really is fifty-three years old. The number forty-eight refers to her risk age. That is, because of her heredity, family health background and personal life-style, Bonnie's chances of dying within the next ten years equal those of the average forty-eight-year-old white woman. If Bonnie alters her life-style as suggested, she will achieve a risk age of forty-six, even as she approaches her fifty-fourth birthday.

The basis of this risk calculation and number juggling is the health hazard appraisal, a technique developed by Lewis C. Robbins, M.D., a former U.S. Public Health Service officer and chief of the Cancer Control Program in Washington, D.C. In 1949, Dr. Robbins devised a health analysis concept that eventually led to the health hazard appraisal. "I thought it should be possible to write a chart for a single individual that would tell his total risk to his health and the degree to which we could decrease that risk by applying preventive measures," says the Indiana physician, who for three years had been involved in setting up the famous Framingham study to monitor the long-term risks and probabilities involved in the development of heart disease. Ten years later, as head of the cancer program, Dr. Robbins had both the opportunity and the funds to put the theory into practice. In 1959, at Temple University, working with public health doctor John Hanlon, M.D., and statistician Harvey Geller, Dr. Robbins conducted the first health-hazard appraisals.

Twenty-five subjects completed the original questionnaires. They described personal living habits, submitted blood and urine samples for laboratory tests and answered questions relating to their own and their families' pasts. The profiles drawn that summer were very simple compared with the detailed analyses that characterize the 1970 health hazard appraisals, but they were a start. Using the assembled data, Dr. Robbins could tell each participant his or her ten most likely causes of death over the next year, the chances of dying from each disease and what steps he or she could take to reduce the risk. (Refinements in the health hazard appraisal would be made in later years, which would enable researchers to pinpoint risk age as well.) The subjects were delighted with the analyses, but Dr. Robbins and his colleagues found they couldn't tell the rest of their profession what they were doing. "We didn't have the right words," he explains. "We called it the health hazard chart, and no one understood what that meant. It was 1962 before we found the term 'prospective medicine.'"

Today, more than 225 public health centers, universities, medical schools, community organizations and private employers provide some version of Dr. Robbins' health hazard appraisal for their target audiences. And thousands of people like Bonnie Simmons are taking advantage of the programs. Today the completed questionnaires are fed into computers rather than tabulated by hand, but the end result remains the same: The health hazard appraisal gives you a chance to see how your health compares with that of other people of your age, sex and race; it tells you what your health risks are—not in general terms but in very specific figures—and it identifies the steps you can take to decrease your risks of disease.

Take Bonnie Simmons, for example. When her firm offered the health risk profiling service at minimal cost to employees, the fifty-three-year-old secretary signed up, mainly out of curiosity. "I wouldn't have wanted to find out about anything immediately life threatening," she admits, "but I also realized you can't hide your head in the sand."

Basically, Bonnie learned that she *is* in pretty good health, that her chances of surviving the next ten years are 28 percent better than average. However, she was informed of the ten most probable causes of death for her in the next decade. These include breast cancer, arteriosclerotic heart disease, lung cancer, cirrhosis of the liver, cancer of the intestines and rectum, and stroke. (The chart on the next page lists the most likely causes of death for men and women ages 55 to 59.)

But Bonnie also was told what she should do if she wants to lower the risk for each risk factor as much as possible, thus attaining her achievable risk age, forty-six. Specific recommendations given to her were as follows: Perform a monthly breast self-examination (this in addition to the annual professional exam she now receives); reduce blood cholesterol level from 210 milligrams to 200 milligrams or less; exercise vigorously (her job, Bonnie says, has made her more sedentary than usual); keep up the no-smoking campaign (she quit smoking one year before participating in the appraisal program); decrease alcohol intake from twelve drinks per week to seven or less; have a protoscopy or rectal examination as her doctor advises and a Hemoccult test, an examination of the stool, at least once every year; reduce salt intake (limiting herself to no more than one teaspoonful per day, unless allowed otherwise by her physician); increase the amount of fruits, vegetables and whole-grained foods in her diet; decrease consumption of saturated fats, processed foods, meat and dairy products; and "greatly reduce" the amount of sweets she consumes.

"Filling out the questionnaire made me conscious of certain things I was doing," says Bonnie Simmons. "I was not aware of how much candy I ate, for example, or how many martinis I drank until I had to answer the questions. I wasn't too crazy about seeing some of this right in front of me on paper."

Ten Major Causes of Death/Ages 55 to 59 Years

White Males
1. Arteriosclerotic heart disease
2. Lung cancer
3. Stroke
4. Cirrhosis of the liver
5. Cancer of the large intestine and rectum
6. Suicide
7. Bronchitis and emphysema
8. Pneumonia
9. Motor vehicle accidents
10. Diabetes mellitus

White Females
1. Arteriosclerotic heart disease
2. Breast cancer
3. Lung cancer
4. Stroke
5. Cancer of the large intestine and rectum
6. Cancer of the ovary
7. Cirrhosis of the liver
8. Diabetes mellitus
9. Rheumatic heart disease
10. Pneumonia

Black Males
1. Arteriosclerotic heart disease
2. Lung cancer
3. Stroke
4. Cirrhosis of the liver
5. Pneumonia
6. Cancer of the large intestine and rectum
7. Cancer of the prostate
8. Cancer of the esophagus
9. Homicide
10. Diabetes mellitus

Black Females
1. Arteriosclerotic heart disease
2. Stroke
3. Breast cancer
4. Diabetes mellitus
5. Lung cancer
6. Cancer of the large intestine and rectum
7. Cirrhosis of the liver
8. Hypertensive heart disease
9. Cancer of the cervix
10. Nephritis and nephrosis

Adapted from PROSPECTIVE MEDICINE. Reprinted with permission of Methodist Hospital of Indiana, Inc.

Already, as a result of her health hazard appraisal, Bonnie has changed some of her living habits. She is walking more. She has stopped adding salt to her food at the table and now uses herbs and spices in its place. She also eats more vegetables (and as a consequence so does her husband). Chicken appears often on the dinner table, but it is rarely fried, unlike before, and Bonnie, a woman who used to "crave meat," now finds that eating it makes her feel too heavy and that she can get by with less. She continues to drink martinis but went on a campaign to educate herself about wine so that she could substitute that for the straight alcoholic drinks.

Her one stumbling block is the breast self-examination. Bonnie is still not conducting the monthly exam, not because she doesn't know the techniques or has any aversion to performing the ritual, but because she just doesn't think of it. Unlike menstruating women, who can link the breast self-examination to their monthly periods, Bonnie, who is postmenopausal, has no regular reminder to associate with the monthly exam. (One physician tells his menopausal patients to use the full moon as a reminder.)

With a slight apology, Bonnie admits that she has started smoking again—she returned to the old habit just before her eldest daughter's wedding. But already she has attended a stop-smoking clinic and insists she's going to quit for good. "The only thing I can't promise is to cut out the candy. My father sold candy, so we always had sweets around the house. I guess it's just one thing I'm too used to."

Bonnie likes the motivation for change she gets from her health hazard appraisal and says she plans to participate in the program regularly. "I'm going to do it again next year, and then I'm going to be able to say, 'I don't smoke anymore. I'm not having as many drinks. I'm doing better.'"

Like Bonnie Simmons, many other middle-aged adults have benefited from health hazard appraisal programs. Faced with a personalized profile of their current health status and with specific suggestions for improving their health, they have made important life-style changes. Examples include:

- A forty-five-year-old woman who consulted her physician about high blood pressure and has faithfully taken her medication ever since.

- A fifty-five-year-old woman who lost thirty-seven pounds and has kept it off.
- A sixty-five-year-old man who now parks his car in the company parking lot as far from the office as possible and walks the extra distance twice daily.
- A middle-aged man who started running for exercise and within one year also stopped smoking.

The health risk profile is valuable because it focuses your attention on the health problems most critical to your well-being. Most of us know that it is not healthy to smoke or drink to excess, for example, but we tend to think that the warnings apply to other people, not to ourselves. A health hazard appraisal profile delivers a personal message. When you can say, "My number-one health risk is lung cancer because my risk is seven times greater than other people's," then you have a better chance of changing your life-style to reduce the risk.

How effective is the health risk profile in prompting healthful life-style changes? Says Dr. Robbins, in the first year after participating in a health risk analysis program, people can lower their risk age as much as four to eight years, although the average is about 1½ years—a significant change for the individuals concerned.

To date, a number of informal studies substantiate these claims. A Canadian study found that, among patients who participated in health hazard appraisals, four out of five made important life-style changes. In Tucson, Arizona, 76 percent of health hazard appraisal participants lowered their risk age after receiving their personalized profiles. In another survey in Moffett Field, California, 107 people were followed for a twelve-month period. When they first took the health risk analyses, the average risk ages of the subjects were about one month less than their real ages. One year later, the average was 1.4 years *below* actual age.

It is important to realize, however, that, when you make suggested life-style changes, you cannot expect the risks for the many different diseases to decrease at similar rates. How much your own risk is altered varies according to the disease. For example, if you quit smoking, your risk of coronary heart disease drops almost immediately, but your risk of lung cancer decreases at a slower rate.

There are no guarantees that taking the health risk profile and making important life-style changes will prevent illness from occurring, but they can help weigh the odds in your favor. "With health risk profiling, we are saying, 'This is what is likely to happen at some time in the future if you don't begin to make some changes,' " says Charles Ross, M.D., of San Diego, California, one of the first physicians in the nation to use computers in the health analysis program. "We can't promise that a disease won't occur anyway, but we can say that it is less likely to develop." Meanwhile, as you implement suggested life-style changes, you reap a second, immediate and tangible benefit: You feel better. That is the reward for everyone, including the fifty-year-old adult. You are taking positive steps to improve your own health. You are doing something that might very well have an impact on your life five, ten or fifteen years from today, and you are going to feel good while you are doing it. "I know, I'm fifty-four," says Dr. Ross. "I've been the ulcer route and the workaholic route. Today I follow the recommendations of my health risk profile. I lead a more healthful life and I feel great. I take time for the things that are important to me."

Health risk profiling is available both for groups and for individuals. Cost to the participants ranges from a few dollars to about twenty-five dollars and varies depending on the sponsoring agency, the number of participants and the profiling center. For information on obtaining an individual profile or on group projects in your area, call your personal physician, your employee medical department, university medical center, public health office or the public information office of a large local hospital or medical society.

Health hazard appraisal is not a perfected science. Risk factors must be periodically updated and the new data incorporated into available programs. Despite these limitations, the health risk profile remains a potentially powerful health education tool when properly used. As with any other health service, you should check the credentials of the sponsoring agency before you commit yourself or your group to a particular health risk analysis program.

Toward a Healthier Environment

Robert F. Allen, Ph.D., wants you to live a healthier life in a healthier world. The fifty-two-year-old psychologist—a former director of special projects for the Ford Foundation and since 1965 president of the Human Resources Institute in Morristown, New Jersey—believes that the most effective way to improve your health is to alter, in specific fashion, the environment that surrounds you and pervades every aspect of your existence. Dr. Allen advocates cultural change—in the family, the school, the workplace and the community. He argues that the only way to help the individual change is to make changes in these areas.

Dr. Allen's ideas are not ivory-tower theories. They were developed in New York ghettos, where he worked with juvenile delinquents and watched as the teenagers repeatedly moved from delinquency to reform and back to delinquency again, despite the best efforts of those trying to redirect the youngsters. Dr. Allen reasoned that, to help the youths he was counseling, he had to give them something to go back to other than the environment that was initially responsible for their induction into a life of petty crime and gang warfare. He began to experiment with creating alternative support systems that in effect changed the environment in which the youngsters lived. By doing so, he helped reduce delinquency by 70 percent among those with whom he worked.

Since then, Dr. Allen has counseled other groups, from Florida migrant workers to urban officials, and has helped them develop effective ways to make large-scale changes in life-styles and attitudes. The same basic ideas that he used to help these people can help all of us in almost every aspect of our lives, he reasons, especially in the area of health. Here Dr. Allen explains how:

In our culture we face incredible odds when we try to alter our life-style and health habits. Despite our best efforts, many of us will fail in our attempts to change the way we live. Of every 1,000 dieters, only 120 will lose weight and, of these, only two or three will maintain their losses. Only 25 percent who start a heart-disease prevention program will maintain the regimen. Among those who quit smoking, few will continue to abstain for more than six months. The problem is not that we are intrinsically weak-willed; the problem is that, to change, we often have to overcome strong cultural norms that support unhealthy behavior. To help ourselves develop a more healthful life-style, we have to alter the cultural norms that are working against us.

Consider some of the life-style habits our culture accepts as appropriate:

- Serving alcoholic drinks at all social gatherings; having drinks at lunch and other meals; preparing a drink when you return home from work
- Serving rich desserts after meals
- Having coffee and sweet rolls available at the work place for morning and sometimes afternoon breaks
- Sitting in front of the television set for hours every evening and on weekends as well.

We like to think our society is becoming more health conscious, but we haven't really succeeded in breaking away from our negative habits. It is likely that, if someone were to serve nonalcoholic drinks, and only those, at the next party you attended, you would be quite surprised and would remember it for quite some time— because drinking alcoholic beverages is still the norm. Try not serving dessert at your next dinner party or holiday get-together and see what happens. Even if no one wanted dessert, some people would wonder why you did not serve it.

We need to start a health revolution in this country. To begin with, people must internalize the idea that life-style changes can and should be made. They need to believe that change is possible. Then they must get together with others who will be supportive. They must talk with their family, co-workers and friends about the impact our culture has on our behavior. People need to understand that the reason they eat fast-food hamburgers, for example, is not necessarily because they want to and find doing so desirable, but because they are responding to a cultural norm or acceptable behavior.

Next, we need to identify where we are and where we want to be in terms of our own health status. Then, finally, we begin the process of change—as individuals, as members of groups, as members of larger organizations. Within this context—within a large group, within a supportive group, for example—change is easier than if we try to change all by ourselves.

Here is a concrete example of how, together, one group of people changed an important and established part of their tradition. Every Friday evening after service at a synagogue for retired people, the participants put together what is called *Oneg Shabat*, in which the women in the group prepare very elaborate foods and lay them out on a table for everyone else. In attendance were seventy-year-old people, most of them a bit overweight, facing an overwhelming array of tasty and very fattening cakes. One man said, "You can't change 3,000 years of Jewish culture," and yet that is exactly what they wanted to change.

And so they changed.

After our discussions, they decided to keep two thirds of the table the way it was, but to set up one third with different kinds of low-calorie foods—fruits and fruit juices, salads, and so on. The people kept track of the amount of these low-calorie, low-fat foods on the table and increased the amounts of those foods as needed. In the meantime, the women attended cooking classes to learn how to prepare these "new" kinds of foods and how to make them as attractive as the cakes had been. It worked. At last report, the "low sugar" end of the table comprised 65 percent of the food served.

So change, real change, had been made. But only after the people involved realized that they could change the cultural norms that dictated how they lived and worked together to do so.

Now consider the cultural norms or accepted behavior patterns that affect your life. If you are a fairly typical white-collar working American, you probably begin your day with either no breakfast, just a cup of coffee, or with too much breakfast—three eggs, bacon, toast and coffee. You drive to work alone or in a car pool. You don't use your seat belt because you haven't the time to put it on or because, in a car pool, someone is sitting on the belt and you don't want to ask him or her to move. You are late for work; traffic is heavy. You may take risks in driving, so that you arrive at work agitated and tense. At work, you reach for the coffee and rolls a co-worker has thoughtfully provided. All morning you sit in a meeting. You'd like to get up and stretch, but instead you fidget (imagine someone getting up and stretching during a meeting!). There's a break at 10:00 A.M.—more coffee and rolls. Later you have lunch with the boss. Most likely you'll order a couple of drinks and a heavy meal. In the afternoon, you are groggy. You don't get much work accomplished, and at 5:00 P.M. you stuff a briefcase full of papers to carry home. At home, you have more drinks and a big dinner. You settle into a favorite chair, turn on the television and reach for your briefcase. Your spouse wants to talk, but you haven't the time. You try to work, but can't concentrate. You go to bed worried about how you will meet your deadlines. At some point, before you drift off to sleep, you think to yourself, "I really should get up earlier tomorrow and exercise before leaving for work. But, I cannot. I'd make too much noise and wake up everyone in the house. Besides, the neighbors would laugh if they saw me. Maybe next week."

How can you change your life? Alone, it is not impossible, but very difficult. With others involved, your odds are much better. Imagine how much different your scenario would be if you talked to your spouse, friends and co-workers about life-style changes that would benefit all of you. Here are some changes you could suggest:

• Exercise together. At home, friends or neighbors could get together for a morning walk or run. At noon, ask co-workers to join you in a walk or in a workout session at a local health club or gym.

• Expand the refreshment selection for breaks. Take turns bringing fresh fruit rather than, or in addition to, cakes and sweets. Add fruit drinks, mineral water and decaffeinated coffee to the menu.

• Allow more travel time to get to work in the morning. Suggest that the car pool leave fifteen minutes earlier, so that you can all arrive more refreshed. Let your co-riders know that you want to use your seat belt.

These are simple suggestions, but they can lead to fundamental changes in your well-being. If you make changes like these together with others, you are creating new cultural norms. You are establishing new, more healthful standards of behavior. You are changing the environment in ways that are beneficial for you as well as for the rest of society.

3

COPING WITH EVERYDAY PHYSICAL PROBLEMS

As we grow older, we tend more than ever to associate good health and vigor with youth. Anything that makes us feel out-of-sorts makes us feel "old." Sore feet, an aching back, too little sleep or eyestrain are minor aches and pains, but they can impose unnecessary limitations and detract from our enjoyment of daily living. There are a host of these everyday problems, all with their own solutions. Here are a few suggestions to help ease minor discomforts:

Back Pain

Almost everyone suffers from it at some point. Disabling or persistent pain requires a thorough check by a physician. Temporary discomfort, the familiar sore spot in the lower back or the upper shoulder, is probably life-style related. Your sore back may stem from any combination of the following: being overweight, even by ten pounds; weak abdominal and back muscles; poor posture.

To help your back, try losing weight, exercising, sitting and driving with a cushion at the small of the back and sleeping on your side with the knees slightly bent. Women should also eliminate girdles, heavy shoulder bags and high-heeled shoes.

Insomnia

Sleep tends to become lighter as we grow older. If you are unable to sleep well night after night, check with your physician. You may benefit from one of the many sleep-disorder clinics established throughout the country.

If you have no trouble falling asleep, but occasionally wake later in the night, your problem may be due to stress or to too much alcohol taken during the previous day. Other culprits may include hunger (offset by a light bedtime snack or glass of warm milk), excessive warmth or cold in the sleeping area, caffeine and chronic smoking. In a study at the Pennsylvania State University Sleep Research and Treatment Center, sudden withdrawal from cigarettes was directly linked to a decrease in the time spent awake at night.

While an occasional bout of exercise is not particularly helpful in aiding sleep, regular daily physical activity will help you sleep better on most nights.

Fatigue

If you are listless one day or feeling less than energetic over a particular weekend, you may simply be tired, not really fatigued. Fatigue generally affects one over a longer period of time, several months, for example. Its symptoms include a withdrawal from one's normal activities and social circle and a general decline in functioning. Every area of your life will be affected. Fatigue can stem from physical illness, depression or extended overwork or activity. If you are listless, feel overwhelmed and just don't have the energy for anything, check with your doctor. Chances are you are suffering from fatigue that can be treated. Don't simply ascribe your condition to age and decide to "live with it."

Constipation

At mid-life, you can maintain normal bodily function. There is no evidence to support the popular notion that constipation is an inevitable outcome of aging. Nor is there any scientific proof that a daily bowel movement is necessary for good health. Your body follows its own schedule.

This does not mean that irregularity is a figment of your imagination. Causes might include lack of exercise, stress, gastrointesti-
nal disease or insufficient bulk in the diet. A chronic situation may
require medical attention. Occasional difficulty might be avoided
with exercise and diet change (see Chapter 12 for information on
adding bulk to the diet). Laxatives should be used only occasionally. Overuse of these products can lead to irritation of the intestinal tract and can result in a physiological dependency.

Dental Problems

British researchers at the Royal College of Surgeons have developed a vaccine they claim will eliminate tooth decay for life.
Although not yet approved for human use, the vaccine could be
one of the great breakthroughs in dentistry, as important for the
middle-aged as for the young. Dental cavities are not limited to
children. Even if you are in your fifties, you are susceptible to
cavities and can lose teeth to decay if the process is not halted in
time. Research shows that nearly half of all Americans who reach
age sixty-five have lost most of their teeth. One culprit is tooth
decay, and another is periodontal disease (inflammation of the
gums and tooth sockets). If not treated quickly, periodontal disease will destroy the gum membrane, causing teeth to become
loose. Periodontal disease also leads to chronic infection in the
mouth that can result in tooth loss. To counter the problem, have
dental plaque removed every six months by your dentist and use
dental floss daily. A paste made of baking soda and hydrogen
peroxide helps heal sore gums. Ask your dentist which teeth are
periodontally involved, then, three or four times a day, pack the
paste around these teeth with a round wooden toothpick, flushing
and brushing between each application. You should notice an
improvement in two to three weeks.

If your mouth hurts, you may be clenching and grinding your
teeth at night when you are asleep. The condition may be a
reaction to stress, or you may have temporomandibular joint
(TMJ) disease. Hot moist applications to the area before and after
eating helps reduce the pain, but check with your dentist in all
cases. He or she may cite dental causes or problems with your diet
—both of which can be corrected.

Diminished Vision and Hearing Acuity

You may feel embarrassed seeking remedies for these problems, but in the long run you will be doing yourself a favor. You may not completely avoid loss of optical and auditory acuity as you age, but you can keep the problem from getting worse if you use glasses or a hearing aid. In any case, any vision or hearing difficulty should be checked by a medical specialist.

Although hearing loss usually does not occur until later in life, vision is often affected by the middle years. To see well, the average sixty-year-old needs seven times as much light as a twenty-year-old. To make the most of your sight, decrease night driving (night vision dims as you age) and check your light sources at home and work. If you haven't upgraded your lighting facilities in the past ten or twenty years, you may be putting undue strain on your eyes. For your own comfort, use more lamps and brighter bulbs.

Sore Feet

Considering the fact that you have twenty-six different bones in your feet, it is little wonder they sometimes hurt. One item to pay special attention to is the proper fit of shoes. Foot size can alter with age. If you are wearing the same size today as you were ten or fifteen years ago, you may be crowding your feet unnecessarily. When you buy your next pair of shoes, make the trip to the store at the end of the day. By then your feet will have expanded 8 to 14 percent in size, and you will have a better chance of ensuring a comfortable fit.

Improperly fitted shoes and elastic hose can be a possible cause of corns. When feasible, wear cotton socks. If you buy elastic stockings or panty hose, avoid the "one size fits all" models. These have too much elastic. Instead, buy the size that is right for you. If corns persist, see a foot specialist. You may need minor surgery.

Structural weakness in the foot is the basic cause of bunions, but ill-fitting shoes can also add to the problem. When bunions form, the joints in the big toe are misaligned. To straighten the toe, a wedge of bone must be surgically removed. To compensate for bunions without surgery, try wearing wider shoes or padding the sensitive area.

A note of caution for diabetics and others with poor circulation: Because your feet may be insensitive to temperature extremes, you should avoid soaking them in hot water, to prevent possible scalding. Your feet may also be insensitive to pain from minor cuts and irritations. Never soak your feet in Epsom salts, because the salts may aggravate foot lesions or sores.

Hair and Hair Loss

As we age, the amount of melanin, a pigmented substance, in the hair shaft decreases; thus, hair tends to turn gray. At the same time, the sebaceous glands in the skin produce less natural oil, so the scalp and hair become dry, and the hair loses its sheen. These processes cannot be halted, but the effects can be countered or minimized with hair colorings and conditioners (read labels carefully and avoid products containing peroxide, which makes hair brittle and weak), a well-balanced diet, regular brushing and routine scalp massages. Also avoid excess use of blow dryers and hair dryers.

Some hair loss from the scalp is normal in middle-aged men and women. Balding is more common in men and is generally linked to heredity and hormonal balance. Although hair transplants are a medically approved treatment for male-pattern baldness, the technique is generally not recommended for men in their fifties (see Chapter 13 for a discussion of aesthetic surgery). In some instances, scalp infections can cause or aggravate hair loss. Check with a physician for proper treatment. Usually after age forty, people begin noticing increased hair growth in the nostrils and ears. This is considered normal. Women may also be more susceptible to growth of facial hair during the menopause as hormone balances change. Facial hair can be bleached, plucked or removed by electrolysis. The latter should be done by a licensed electrolysist.

Skin

Beginning around age forty, certain changes begin to affect the skin. Many of these changes have an impact on the deeper layers of the skin, that is, on the dermis and the underlying fatty tissue.

Elasticity in the supporting fibers of the dermis is diminished; sebaceous glands produce less oil, and the dermis may become thinner and less able to retain water. The overall effect of these alterations is wrinkles, dryness and sagging skin.

Factors that aggravate the development of "aging skin" include excessive exposure to sun, wind and hot water. In addition, poor diet, excessive use of alcohol and an overly sedentary life-style may hasten the aging process. To minimize these changes, one should exercise, eat a balanced diet, wear cotton-lined rubber gloves for household and outdoor chores and use emollient (softening) creams when dryness occurs.

The daily application of sunscreen products containing PABA (para-aminobenzoic acid) before going outdoors will reduce cumulative sun damage considerably. PABA blocks the most intense solar ultraviolet rays. People who are bothered by significant wrinkling or sagging skin may consider having plastic surgery (see Chapter 13 for a discussion of aesthetic surgery).

Beyond middle age, people become more susceptible to a variety of skin growths. Some are problematic; others are merely annoying from a cosmetic viewpoint. It may help you to familiarize yourself with the characteristics of the more common growths:

• *Actinic keratoses.* These gritty, wartlike growths, often pinkish-white in color, are found most commonly on the face and hands. They are directly related to sun exposure and, if untreated, may eventually lead to skin cancer. Those affected tend to be fair-skinned and have outdoor occupations or avocations. Actinic keratoses are treated for cosmetic reasons, but also, more importantly, for the prevention of possible skin cancer.

• *Seborrheic keratoses.* These are dark-brown, warty growths that look like they have been stuck onto the skin surface. They can occur singly or in large numbers (as many as forty or fifty), may be pockmarked on the surface and have a somewhat greasy appearance. They are most common on the face and upper trunk, especially the back. These growths are benign and are treated essentially for cosmetic reasons. They should be examined, however, to ensure that they do not represent a more serious type of growth.

• *Sebaceous hyperplasias.* These, too, are benign and are very common in middle-aged and older adults. They are tiny, smooth, yellowish buttonlike growths with a tendency to occur on the forehead and upper face.

• *Telangiectasias.* These are not growths, but are abnormally dilated blood vessels found on the nose, cheeks and forehead. While alcohol can contribute to the problem, those affected are not necessarily heavy drinkers and should not be unfairly labeled as such. Equally important contributing factors are hot beverages of any kind, including tea and coffee, as well as smoking. Treatment is for cosmetic reasons.

• *Papillomas.* These growths, called skin tags, are small fleshy shriveled sacks of skin that protrude abruptly from the surface and tend to occur on the neck, underarm and breast area. They are not medically significant, and treatment is usually for cosmetic reasons.

• *Basal cell carcinomas.* These waxy nodules of varying size are growths that may eventually ulcerate. They are considered to be malignant and are generally associated with chronic overexposure to sunlight. They are also soft to the touch and occur most often on the face. They hardly ever metastasize—that is, spread to other parts of the body—but if left untreated may invade locally and affect adjacent structures. The cure rate is 90 percent or higher if treated early.

• *Squamous cell carcinomas.* These are hard, roughened growths with a warty appearance, usually light in color. They also are often associated with sun exposure, may originate from actinic keratoses and may ulcerate. Again, the face and hands are frequently involved. These are not as common as basal cell carcinomas, but, because they can metastasize, early treatment is essential.

• *Melanomas.* These malignancies develop from moles (or nevi), are usually black mixed with shades of red or blue and may also be associated with sun exposure. Melanomas can occur at any age, but especially beyond age thirty. Common sites are the back, upper chest, face, arms and lower legs. About half develop from previously existing moles and half seem to appear spontaneously. Danger signals include itching, bleeding and any change in color or size.

A number of techniques are available for removing the various skin growths. They can be frozen (cryosurgery), scraped off (curettage), electrocoagulated (destroyed with an electric needle), destroyed with chemical solutions or excised by surgical means. Malignant growths may also be treated with X rays. In general, the treatments are applied in the physician's office.

4

THE FIFTIES: A TIME FOR PERSONAL GROWTH

In 1950, psychoanalyst Erik H. Erikson, then at the University of California, Berkeley and San Francisco, helped create a revolution in the field of human psychology. In *Childhood and Society*, published that year, Erikson summarized nearly twenty years of research that for the first time offered convincing evidence that maturation and personal growth extend well beyond childhood and continue throughout adulthood.

For years, many mental health professionals have been influenced primarily by the work of Sigmund Freud, who stressed the importance of the early years of life. According to Freud's theories, the formative years were the most critical segment of development. Freud believed that, to a very large extent, the experiences of childhood determined adult character structure and vulnerabilities. The child, in effect, was accepted as the father of the man.

Given the luxury of hindsight, we can criticize Freud's approach to personality development as being too limited. But, when we look at the environment in which Freud worked, we see that this criticism is unwarranted. For one thing, Freud lived in a very different world than we do today. The average life span during his time was less than fifty years. By our standards, adulthood was a relatively short and inflexible period. In fact, few people paid serious attention to later life. The science of psychology itself was in relative infancy. There was no such thing as "life-span" theory.

The concept of developmental psychology did not even exist. Freud began his work as a pioneer in the field. We can see now that his efforts were only a beginning, albeit an important one, in the understanding of human growth and development.

Erikson challenged Freud's premise about the dominant influence of the early years and helped to develop the concept of life cycles and continued growth. Since the 1950s, other studies have substantiated and expanded upon Erikson's work. The overall result is a radical shift in the way psychiatrists and psychologists view adult development.

"In the past we had a tendency to view psychological change, like physiological change, as fate," explains George Maddox, Ph.D., director of the Center for the Study of Aging and Human Development at Duke University Medical Center, Durham, North Carolina. "Now we have come to the position that we can just possibly change things ourselves, psychologically as well as physically. Change must be viewed realistically. But at least change is now recognized as a possibility for adults."

As adults, we are freed from the chains that might make us subservient to our past. But we are also charged with a new responsibility. In uncovering evidence of growth and of the continuing unfolding and development of the human psyche, the men and women who study life's various stages discovered that to a large extent it is the individual who makes the difference between fulfillment and despair. Life's many circumstances are important and play a part, of course, but the instrument for growth, change and development lies within the self.

To date, our understanding of adult psychological development is far from complete. Little attention has been paid to the cultural and ethnic factors that can have an impact on people's lives. Studies of women lag far behind those of men. And critics point out that rapid societal changes dictate the need for continual updating of life-span theories.

Nonetheless, the underlying idea, first suggested by Erikson, remains unchallenged—that people can grow and change throughout their adult lives. The concept of adult psychological growth is a revolutionary idea. It can have an important and positive impact on your life during the fifties decade. But personal growth does not occur unaided. You affect the process.

To a very great extent, you can stimulate growth or hamper it.

Daniel J. Levinson, Ph.D., has been actively studying adult psychological development for nearly two decades. He is professor of psychology at the Yale University School of Medicine, New Haven, Connecticut, and author of *The Seasons of a Man's Life* (Alfred A. Knopf, Inc., 1978). Dr. Levinson offers the following observations:

• To stimulate psychological growth during your middle years, you must be sure that your life has substance and purpose.

The quest for meaning is essential to well-being throughout life. It is as important now as ever. No matter how much money or fame or power you have, these are not enough to ensure a sense of self-worth. If you are to live with intensity and enthusiasm, you need to measure yourself by more than the external criteria of success used by society. If you are to feel satisfied with life and to continue to grow and develop as an adult, you need an existence that is meaningful.

People can be content with their lives even if they lack a sense of intrinsic worth. But they enjoy their contentment at the cost of any real involvement. Chances are their lives become trivial and very limited. Instead of growth, they experience stagnation. It is a choice all of us make.

To grow, you must feel that your life has value, both for yourself and for other people. You need a purpose, a "reason for living." What gives purpose to your existence at age fifty may be different from what provided meaning at an earlier age, but this is only natural. Your goals can and will change.

• To experience growth and enrichment in the middle years, you need to recognize and to pursue the special opportunities that middle age offers.

During mid-life, we are freed internally to become uniquely individual, we can begin to lessen the hold society has on us. We are able to separate personal goals and ambitions from those created by society. We can listen to the inner voice that defines who and what we are. We begin setting our own standards and living according to them. This is a process called individuation. It allows us to become more creative, more reflective and more understanding of ourselves and others.

At the same time, middle age provides the opportunity to excel externally. Increased understanding of how the world works and greater self-confidence allow us to become leaders in society and in the workplace. Unless our lives are hampered in some special way, most of us can become senior members in our particular worlds—politics, science, education, the arts, business and in all social institutions. We assume a great responsibility for our own work and for the work of others; we can take a larger role in shaping and directing the current generation of young adults. We have, in short, an opportunity to make our mark upon the world in which we live.

• To ensure continued psychological growth through the fifties, we must learn to take advantage of change.

As we go through life, we will experience many changes. Changes occur whether we wish them to or not. The crux of the matter is not whether we avoid change, but whether we make change work for the better. The responsibility rests largely with each of us. Choices must be made, and bets must be placed. You must decide, "This I will settle for; this I will work for."

The fifties present their own special problems. But there is more to mid-life than dilemmas. If you are willing to grow, you can make the fifties an extremely satisfying decade of life.

Growth in the Middle Years: One Woman's Experience

Sheila Grant was a lively, intelligent young girl, the third of four daughters. She was reared in the suburbs of Minneapolis, under the guidance of a strict but loving father and a shy, undemanding mother.

Like her sisters, Sheila was allowed the usual rebelliousness of youth. Full crinolines and light lipstick were permitted at age sixteen. However, enlisting in the armed forces, something she wanted to do, was forbidden at age eighteen. Instead, at her father's direction, Sheila attended junior college. With his permission, she married at age twenty-two.

Within three years, Sheila and her husband, Alan, had two small sons and a modest home in the country. Their roles were clearly delineated. Alan, an independent insurance broker, was to be the breadwinner. Sheila was to be the wife and mother.

Sheila gave Alan the moral and social support he needed to

make his business a success. The rest of her energy she devoted exclusively to her children and to the home. Sheila Grant was den mother, church mother, library volunteer and weekend camper for her sons. Her home was spotless; her meals were always on schedule.

For a brief period, when money was scarce, Sheila took a part-time job outside the home, asking Alan's permission first. Later, with the birth of a third child, a daughter, she again enthusiastically embraced the role of mother and homemaker.

From the beginning of her marriage, Sheila had longed for adult friends but had avoided all but the most superficial relationships with the women she knew. "I grew up believing that you shared your intimate thoughts only with your husband," she explains. "When you talked with friends, it was only to exchange pleasantries."

In the eyes of society, says Sheila, she was always a good wife and mother. In her own mind, however, she was an insecure, immature woman haunted by the subconscious fear that if she did not measure up to an imaginary standard of perfection, her husband, a former Navy officer, would leave her. (The threat originated not with Alan but with Sheila's own mother. "He'll never stay with you," the older woman had warned just before her daughter's wedding. "He's a sailor and he has to have a girl in every port.")

Throughout most of her early adult life, says Sheila, she lived by two basic tenets. One decreed that control of her life rested with her husband; the other that people were psychologically immutable. "Alan did not demand responsibility for my life," she says. "I gave it to him. I thought that was expected. Later, when I tried to change him and could not, I decided no one could be changed, and I included myself in that view, too."

Sheila Grant viewed life as a series of unalterable situations that she had no choice but to accept. She found her refuge in conforming to external standards. Sheila survived by doing the expected. She avoided problems by feigning confusion. She never questioned; she never formed opinions. "If I was unhappy at home, it was my husband's fault. If I was dissatisfied with something in the community, I thought, 'Well, that's life.' And I never expressed anger because I thought that nice girls didn't do that."

Looking back on this period that stretched from early to middle adulthood, Sheila says simply, "I stopped growing as a person. I don't know if I thought I couldn't or shouldn't keep developing myself, but in any case I did not do it."

Then, when Sheila Grant was forty-seven years old, she underwent a hysterectomy. She had barely recovered from the operation when both her mother-in-law and her father-in-law died. Several months later, she and Alan sold their home and moved to a different city. Shortly afterward, Alan was diagnosed as having cancer.

"I think I could have dealt with everything else if Alan hadn't become ill," says Sheila. "But his illness was devastating. It unleashed the horror of my unspoken fear that someday he would leave me, and it completely overshadowed everything else that had happened. How can you even think of other problems when your husband has cancer? How can you be concerned about anyone but him without feeling immensely selfish and shameful?"

Alan responded well to surgery and subsequent therapy and recovered from his disease. But Sheila was overwhelmed by the events that had overtaken her life. She became emotionally immobilized. She withdrew into a shell. "For nearly two years I kept my mind and emotions locked in a box. I cooked and did laundry and went to church, but it was like there was no me," she explains. "I was not really aware of anything that happened."

All the while, though, an incredible rage was building inside Sheila. "It was anger at myself for not being able to cope," she says.

Sheila's anger finally came to the surface when her two eldest children were in college. Suddenly Sheila saw her offspring doing what she had never allowed herself to do. They challenged life head-on; they solved problems; they questioned; they struggled to maintain personal standards that were sometimes different from the norm.

"I saw them grow and I was envious," says Sheila. "I wanted some of that for myself, too, and with their encouragement I began looking for something more out of life."

For Sheila, the next few years were tumultuous. She attended community and church-sponsored discussion and therapy sessions, first alone and then with her husband. She took a part-time job working in a dentist's office and shortly afterward became involved in local politics. She shed the cloak of shyness that she had used as a defense mechanism and sought out friendships with other women. She discarded her former "too confused to cope" stance and began learning to deal with her problems, one step at a time. For a period she was, by her own admission, overbearing, but this passed.

Today, says Sheila Grant, she is a different person at age fifty-seven than she was ten years ago. "I learned that I could change," she explains. "I learned that I could have my own thoughts and that they could be different from someone else's. I learned that my husband and family loved me even if I made mistakes and had my faults. I recognized that my life offered options, a possibility I never even considered before. I discovered I could have control over my own existence and that I could be responsible for my own happiness. I would say that my life has become 1,000 times more exciting."

As for the future? "I feel good about it," says Sheila Grant. "That's part of what I learned: I can survive. I can change. I can grow."

5

THE MYTHS OF THE
MID-LIFE CRISIS

Despite media coverage and popular notions to the contrary, there is more good news than bad to report about the event known as the "mid-life crisis."

The concept itself is relatively new in the field of mental health. It is not completely understood, and much more investigation is needed before final conclusions can be drawn. Nonetheless, the findings to date are encouraging. Enough factual data have accumulated to allow us to discuss the realities in a reasonable fashion and to refute the misconceptions that have developed.

Basically, there are three major myths concerning psychological crisis in the middle years.

Myth 1. The majority of middle-aged men and women can expect to undergo serious psychological crises during mid-life.

In fact, there are no data to substantiate this claim. The studies that have been conducted to date tend to disprove the theory that mid-life crisis is a universal or widespread event.

For example, an interim report on a twenty-year follow-up study of more than 200 middle-aged employees of the Bell Telephone system revealed that only a minority—22 percent of the subjects who had participated in the study—were experiencing a mid-life crisis. Among middle-aged women surveyed in a study conducted by psychologists from the Wellesley College Center for Research on Women, only 12 percent reported dissatisfaction with their lives.

"We ought to bury the notion of universal, age-related life crisis," concluded researchers who recently conducted the Colchester Study of Aging in England. According to the British report, "Many people *never* [italics added] experience any discernible psychological crisis."

What people *do* experience and share during the middle years are transition stages, in which both men and women move into other, different phases of life: Women experience menopause; working adults prepare for retirement; some people contemplate career changes; parents witness their children leaving home and most people encounter at least minor changes in sexual and general physiological functioning. For many members of society, mid-life is a time when conflicts develop because the boundaries of traditional sex roles begin to blur and become less well defined. During middle age it is also not unusual to experience the death of a parent, spouse or peer.

Each of these life changes demands adaptation and adjustment. But this does not mean that any one of them must result in a psychological crisis. Just because you experience change, disappointment or trauma during your middle years does not mean you will undergo a mid-life crisis.

Myth 2. Life crises occur only during the middle years.

This hypothesis is also not true. Crises can occur at any time during our lives. There are, in fact, indications that for many adults the early years are much more stressful than the middle years.

There are identifiable periods in life when circumstances increase the potential for psychological problems or adjustment and adaptation. Adolescence is one such period. Mid-life is another. But this does not mean that every adolescent or every middle-aged adult experiences crisis. Nor does it mean that crises do not develop at other stages of life. The term *mid-life crisis* itself is misleading, because it implies that crisis is a function of a particular age period. This has been proven to be false.

Unfortunately, mid-life crisis has become a popular label, one that is often used to cover up or explain away potentially serious problems. How often have you heard people say, "It's just a crisis phase. It will pass." They dismiss the complaints of an unhappy spouse, a co-worker's bizarre behavior or their own anxieties rather than to try to understand their feelings and discern the root of personal or interpersonal problems.

Even researchers who pioneered the study of the mid-life crisis warn about potential abuses of the phrase. There is the very real danger that discussion of mid-life crises disintegrates into "cock-tail-party chatter." Or that people use the term to excuse irresponsible and perhaps immature behavior, saying, "I'm having a mid-life crisis, so I can do whatever I want to do."

Myth 3. Certain life events cause psychological crises, and the middle-aged individual who experiences these events or traumas cannot avoid undergoing a mid-life crisis.

This is a popular notion, but it is not true.

In fact, there is no universal cause-and-effect relationship between specific life events and a psychological crisis. Crisis is not only a consequence of a particular situation; it is often the result of an individual's response to an event.

For example, one parent may feel depleted by the departure of children from the home, whereas another may view the change as an opportunity for personal development. Job loss may represent a devastating blow to one individual, whereas it may become a blessing in disguise to another.

For a life crisis to occur, both a precipitating event or stimulus *and* a noncoping response must be present. People who are in crisis usually experience bouts of sadness; they may feel moderately depressed; they may become withdrawn, resentful or angry. Often, relationships with family members, co-workers and friends are negatively affected. These are all possible manifestations of an individual's inability to deal with a particular problem or to adjust to a specific event occurring in his or her life. Thus, by our definition, mid-life crisis can be described as any severe and urgent problem people face during the middle years that causes or results in marked changes in how they feel about themselves and/or how they relate to their surroundings. Such crises, to repeat, are by no means inevitable; there *are* ways to avoid them.

David L. Gutmann, Ph.D., professor of psychiatry and behavioral science at Northwestern University Medical School, in Chicago, recommends that adults consciously try to recognize and anticipate the risks and changes inherent in the middle years. By knowing what changes to expect and by preparing themselves psychologically for these events *before* they occur, you can minimize your chances of experiencing them as a crisis.

What can you do if a psychological crisis occurs at mid-life? Suggests Dr. Gutmann:

• First, look for the root of the problem. This may not be simple to determine. Oftentimes pinpointing the source of your distress may require frank and arduous discussions with individuals trained to hear you out. Sometimes family members and friends may be helpful.

• Second, if you are able to identify the cause of your troubles, think about your options. Determine the responses available to you and decide which are rational and which are irrational. Doing so will help you put the problem into focus and help you deal with it realistically.

A true mid-life crisis is indeed statistically rare. However, a full-blown crisis is not a minor matter. It can entail alcoholism, erratic behavior and even suicidal depression. It should be taken seriously, and reasonable forms of treatment should not be ruled out. However, what is encouraging to note, says Dr. Gutmann, is that most of us *do* surmount stresses fairly well. Most of us will not face a serious crisis at mid-life.

The View from the Middle: Lives Without Crises

"I feel that this is my time for reaping rewards from life," says fifty-two-year-old Connie Malloy. "I have worked hard all my life and prepared for this period. Now I want to enjoy it."

Connie Malloy works in the purchasing department of a large international firm. Her husband, Walter, age fifty-three, is a locomotive engineer. He has been employed by the same company for more than thirty years. The Malloys have two married sons, an extensive network of longtime friends and a myriad of social and recreational activities that they pursue either together or individually. "I feel that my life is very full," says Connie. "We are not wealthy people, but we are comfortable, and within reason we can do what we want. We have what is most important to us—our health and our friends."

Fate has not always been kind to Connie. During her early married years, she lived on an economic shoestring and defied a then more-conservative society that harshly criticized marriage between persons of different religions. Later Connie endured two unsuccessful pregnancies, losing the daughters she had always hoped for. More recently she saw her mother through a long and unsuccessful bout with cancer. Still, Connie endured and triumphed, slowly realizing the dreams and goals she had set: a home of her own, paid for; a college education for her sons; a marriage that remains strong.

At mid-life, Connie Malloy is vigorous and dynamic. She is sensitive to her own needs as well as to those of others; she is attuned to life and change. Connie focuses her attention not on what the world has denied her but on the promise that it continues to hold.

"I believe you have to accept the fact that you can't have everything you want, either in a material or in a spiritual sense," she explains. "And I think you have to realize that no one escapes tragedy in life, that the world is not being unfair if everything doesn't work out the way you want it to. I have always had goals, and I will always want to have something to strive for, but I try to be realistic and fit my goals to my life, as well as vice versa."

For Connie, the bottom line is accepting personal responsibility for one's own life. "In a sense I feel lucky that my life is as good as it is," she says. "But I also know that I am a very determined person and that I would do whatever was necessary to change things if I weren't satisfied. I sincerely believe that you have to make the effort to be happy. Life is too short not to enjoy it."

At a time in life when many people anticipate personal crises, Connie Malloy is confident and optimistic. She is comfortable with her role and pleased with, rather than threatened by, her increasing years. "Middle age agrees with me," says Connie Malloy, echoing a sentiment being heard more often throughout the country. "Maybe I'd like to make a few minor improvements, but basically I wouldn't change myself for the world. I like who I am and what I am."

"I am amazed that I am as old as I am," says John Rose, a

fifty-one-year-old West Coast businessman. "I don't believe it. I don't feel it. If someone had told me fifteen years ago that my life would be as good as it is now, I would have laughed. I thought that at age fifty life became negative. My life has never been better."

For John, middle age is not a time of crisis but rather a period of great calm. "When I was younger, I went through long periods of insecurity, during which I questioned my value as a person and worried constantly about the future. Now I have more confidence in myself. I have a sense of pride in my accomplishments and a sense of reassurance that comes from knowing I have solved problems in the past and will be able to continue to do so in the future."

A stint as a fighter pilot in the Korean conflict, an unhappy marriage at home and years of hard work establishing his own business have left him with few delusions about life and about himself. "I may not always like life and who I am," he says, "but I think I have a better understanding of things now. I have learned to keep myself in focus."

Does he fear change? No, says John. "Why should I? I have been facing it for fifty years. I know that unless I am willing to do something about a situation, then it is not going to change. I know what has happened in the past, but that is all gone. If something is ever going to happen again, it is going to happen now."

The solution to life, says John Rose, is to recognize that you have to take care of yourself, both physically and emotionally.

"Address your problems to the mirror," he advises. "I have seen too many people who reach this point in life and suddenly start to blame all their problems on their age. Rather than strive for what they can accomplish, they use age as an excuse for giving up and doing nothing.

"But I have also seen the opposite, people who are marvelous and vital well into their later years."

That contrast, says John, has taught him an important lesson. "You don't quit playing the game because you get old; you get old because you quit playing."

As for himself, says John, "I'm really rather proud of being in my fifties. I hope other people feel the same way."

6

EASING THE STRESSES AND STRAINS OF MID-LIFE

To everything there is a season, and a time to every purpose under the heaven.

Ecclesiastes 3:1

"Every season has its own time; it is important in its own right and needs to be understood in its own terms," writes Yale University professor Daniel J. Levinson, Ph.D., in *The Seasons of a Man's Life*.

What, then, are the terms of the middle years? Says Dr. Levinson, on the one hand, middle age is about growth, about living fully and about becoming more of a person. Any discussion of the middle years would be incomplete without taking account of these concerns. On the other hand, he explains, middle age is also about getting older and suffering losses. It is facing the dilemmas that have to do with this particular season of life.

Not everyone shares the same problems in middle age. To a large extent, the circumstances of life are dictated by a variety of factors that are different for each of us. But middle age, like other periods, also claims its own special issues.

In this chapter, we will look at several problem areas that are concerns for people who are in their fifties. The issues involve questions of personal mortality and regrets, the experience of stress at mid-life and depression.

The issues are intrinsically complex. At times they can also be cloaked with myth and clouded by unrealistic fears. But they are not insurmountable. The problems you may face during the middle years are often problems with very real solutions.

Psychological Issues of the Fifties

During mid-life, the passage of time becomes an issue difficult to avoid. The surrounding world provides an onslaught of both subtle and obvious reminders. Children enter college, marry or take a first job; a son or daughter beats you at a game of tennis; a colleague retires; you spend an evening viewing family slides or snapshots and see undeniable proof of your own aging process. At mid-life you become aware of a change in perspective.

GROWING OLDER IN A YOUTH-ORIENTED SOCIETY

Suddenly, it seems, you are in the middle. You can simultaneously look forward and backward. Inexorably, you realize that the balance of your life is shifting between the number of years lived and the number of years left to live. Yet, at the same time, you live in a society that judges people by what they do, how much money they earn and what kind of future they have. Because the middle-aged have less future than the young, they are less valued. This is a pervasive trend that is difficult to counter and that can generate negative psychological pressures.

How can you learn to deal with the conflicts that arise? First, realize that you have certain factors in your favor. As a group, increased numbers, better health and greater financial resources give your generation advantages denied previous generations of middle-aged adults. Also, researchers note that there are a number of adaptive measures you can utilize to counter the pressures of a society that dotes on the young and to ensure continued self-esteem and satisfaction with life. Their suggestions include:

• Learning to rely more heavily on internal rather than external measures of self-worth. This means, for example, valuing yourself for your knowledge and expertise, rather than for your bank account or job title. In another chapter we talked about personal psychological growth and the process of individuation; both can be critical to maintaining personal prestige. They allow you and not society to determine what is important in your value system and to control your life.

• Utilizing untapped personal resources. You probably have talents and abilities that have lain dormant during the busy years of establishing a career and rearing a family. These resources have not disappeared; they have simply been forgotten. By rediscovering them, you enrich yourself; you create new perspectives and possibilities.

• Developing a rich and complex sense of self. At mid-life, changes begin to occur over which you have no control. If your sense of self is simply concerned with maintaining a youthful appearance, you will in a sense be defenseless against these changes and their effects. But if your sense of self encompasses what you have accomplished and what you have been, if it involves past relationships that have enriched you, if your sense of self includes enjoyment and curiosity about life, then it can help defend you against the pressures of society and time.

Finally, and most importantly, you need to realize that you must assume responsibility for your role in and your approach to life. You alone can determine the attitudes and the ideals by which you will live.

"I guess the trick is to get the good of your experience without lapsing into the tiresome view that everything has happened twenty times before, so what's the big deal?" says magazine columnist Meg Greenfield. "I have convinced myself of this," she says. "The important thing is not what others think about your advancing age or even what you think of it yourself—but rather what and how you think about the world outside you."

DEALING WITH REGRETS AND DISAPPOINTMENTS

During the middle years most of us must face the issue of regrets and unrealized dreams. It is important to realize that while you cannot escape from having some unfulfilled expectations, you can learn to deal effectively with unrealized dreams. By doing so, you help ensure a sense of personal satisfaction and fulfillment for both the present and the future.

First of all, you should dismiss the idea that serious regrets are a common problem for most people during the middle years. This is simply not true. Researchers find that the concept of regrets, especially as it is associated with specific career choices, is not even relevant for a large portion of society. We have a myth in our culture that says that, at age fifty, people face the possibility they may never get to be chairman of the board, but this is really an issue for only a small segment of society. It does not even enter into the realities of most people.

For most of us, doubts and regrets are not pervasive and over-whelming. Rather, they are expressed as nagging reminders of goals we once set and, for whatever reasons, did not fulfill. Most of us express our regrets in simple terms: I should have done X, or I wish I had done Y. These doubts do not represent serious traumas, but if we do not learn to cope with them, we can let them grow out of proportion. How can we deal with these old dreams? Here are some suggestions:

First, separate your unfulfilled dreams from the unfulfilled dreams imposed on you by your parents or spouse. It is sometimes surprising how many regrets we suffer that are not of our own making. Who is disappointed that you became an artist instead of an engineer—you or your father? Who regrets that you lost the bid for sheriff in your county—you or your spouse? By distin-guishing between *your* unrealized dreams and the unrealized dreams prescribed by others, you may be able to free yourself from much unnecessary guilt.

Second, determine if your unrealized goals represent realistic goals or are really the products of a flight of fancy or wishful thinking. Could you really have been a top model in New York or war correspondent if you hadn't married your high school sweetheart? Could you really have become a millionaire by age thirty-five if you had only worked harder? Too often we punish ourselves because we have not achieved goals that never were within our grasp. We create unrealistic dreams, then suffer un-necessary guilt because we did not live up to them. This is emo-tional baggage we should shed at mid-life.

Next, ask yourself, honestly, Is this really important to me? Does it matter at this point in my life that I went to X university rather than to Y? Does it matter that I did not complete my postgraduate work, that I was not accepted in officers training school, that I was fired from my first job? Some disappointments are painful; these we must face. But we should also realize that other past events have little or no relevancy in our current lives and that we can relieve ourselves of the emotional burdens of worrying about those events.

If you have identified unrealized expectations that remain important to you, ask yourself, What can I do about them now? In some instances, you may simply have to accept the fact that a situation cannot be changed—no matter how hard you try or how much you wish it could be altered. But in many other cases you can resurrect old dreams and take steps now to fulfill former expectations. In Chapter 15 we shall see many examples of people who have successfully and happily redirected their lives in the pursuit of goals they had previously abandoned. It is very possible that you may be able to do the same for yourself.

Finally, remember that it is important to avoid taking your regrets out of context. It is much better, instead, to balance your disappointments with your successes. Each of us has a reservoir of past events and achievements we can draw upon to shape our present identities. Rather than focus your thoughts on what you did not accomplish, think of all the things you have done and of how important the accomplishments are to you, your family and your community. Give yourself credit for integrity, for diligence, for the happiness you have brought to others; remember all the obstacles you have overcome, all the problems you have solved. In all likelihood you will discover that your unrealized dreams are more than outweighed by the very real achievements of your life.

FACING THE ISSUE OF PERSONAL MORTALITY

More than a decade ago, British psychoanalyst Elliott Jacques labeled death "the central and crucial feature of the mid-life phase." But he also said, "We can live with it, without an overwhelming sense of persecution." Modern research substantiates Jacques' observations. Say researchers, it is a myth that death creates immense anxiety for the middle-aged. For most of us, it is not a debilitating subject; rather it is an issue that we are able to face and with which we learn to cope.

We deal with our own theoretical deaths just as we deal with the actual death of a loved one. We grieve. We mourn our own loss of youth. We experience periods of denial, anger, sadness and finally acceptance. When we reach this final stage, we have come to terms with the issue of personal mortality, and death ceases to be problematic.

What is critical is that we not try to deny the fact of personal mortality. Instead we must develop positive coping mechanisms that allow us to accept the fact of our eventual death.

How do other middle-aged men and women face the issue of personal mortality? In numerous surveys, University of Chicago researcher Morton A. Lieberman, Ph.D., has asked the aged about their views on death. On the basis of their responses, we see that most people utilize one of three approaches in facing the reality of personal mortality.

First, many people are able to accept death because of their religious faith. They view death as a means of spiritual fulfillment. For them death provides the opportunity to reap a heavenly reward. Second, others view death as the logical balance to life. They feel they have lived a good and happy existence and thus have no reason to fear death. Finally, the majority of aged adults simply identify with the flow of life. They consider death part of the life process. Through our deaths, they say, we make way for the next generation to carry on.

We can use any or all of these approaches, or we can develop our own personal philosophies to help ourselves face and accept the reality of personal mortality. Whatever gives you comfort, whatever makes it easier for you to deal with this issue in a way that is not psychologically disruptive is the right way for you, says Dr. Lieberman. For all of us the issue of mortality remains a highly personal matter. We face the issue at mid-life, we resolve it and we go on.

Coping with Stress

In field surveys and medical laboratories, researchers continue seeking answers to the complex questions raised by the issue of psychological stress. To date, findings are both inconclusive and sometimes contradictory. There are, for example, studies that identify mid-life as a period of increased emotional and psychological stress. There are other studies that conclude that the middle-aged are not subject to more stress than are people in other age groups. One school of thought suggests that certain changes or key events that occur during one's life, such as pending retirement and departure of children, are by nature stressful. Another argues that these events cause stress only when they occur unexpectedly or at the "wrong time" in the life cycle. One body of evidence supports the idea of a cause-and-effect relationship between stress and physical illness; another maintains that no hard proof exists to support this theory. We are, unfortunately, still at a stage in the research on stress where much more information is needed. We cannot make definitive statements about all aspects of stress. But this does not mean that we cannot say anything.

Much is known about stress and its general impact on physical, emotional and psychological well-being. Much of the existing knowledge about stress applies directly to people in middle age.

Stress is anything that puts strain on your life. Psychological stress can be defined as any pressure that demands an unusual response. The response can be physiological or emotional or both; it can be fleeting or prolonged. Stress itself can be a positive or a negative force, although the term is used more commonly, as it is here, to denote the latter.

Certain factors that can contribute to stress are characteristic of different life periods. This does not mean that everyone in a particular age group experiences the same kinds of stress. In mid-life, for example, the psychological issues of aging may present a problem for one person while, for another, alienation from children or job dissatisfaction may be a principal factor for stress. It is a myth to think that because you are middle-aged, you necessarily face a prepackaged compendium of problems labeled mid-life stress factors. What causes stress for you may be specific to your ethnic and socioeconomic background and will be affected by your sex, marital status and occupation.

It is important that you learn to identify specific sources of stress. This is an essential step in learning to deal with them. Stress may be caused by internal turmoil. It can also stem from external factors. Economic difficulties, community problems and even societal changes are among the external factors that can impinge upon your life in a stressful fashion. "We have found that most of the issues confronting people in the middle years are, in fact, social rather than internal," says Paul T. Costa, Jr., Ph.D., chief of the Section on Stress and Coping in the Laboratory of Behavioral

Sciences, at the National Gerontology Research Center in Baltimore, Maryland. "We see people who are dealing with fifty years worth of memories, values and traditions while at the same time they are confronting a chaotic world that changes by the hour—a situation that can produce enormous stress."

Anything you do in response to the factors causing stress is called coping. Coping is an attempt to maintain equilibrium and balance in the face of buffeting forces. Coping mechanisms can be conscious or unconscious, passive or active. They may be designed either to solve problems or to deal with the emotional turmoil that conflicts produce. Coping mechanisms may also be positive or negative, depending upon their effectiveness and their physical and psychological impact on the individual who is experiencing stress.

How many coping mechanisms exist? Several years ago, a National Institutes of Health study identified seventeen different coping strategies. These included seeking advice, being self-assertive and making positive comparisons, such as "We're all in the same boat," to de-emphasize your own unhappiness. But, the study noted, the responses cited represent only a portion of the full range of coping mechanisms adults actually employ in dealing with life's problems.

A study on coping involving some 2,000 Chicago adults suggests that coping responses can be divided into three major categories: (1) facing one's problems and taking direct action to solve them, (2) rationalizing one's situations ("I can't do anything about it anyway") and avoiding dealing with painful issues and (3) simply accepting one's lot and making no attempts to alter a stress-inducing environment. Interestingly, the subjects in the study tended to utilize all three kinds of coping mechanisms interchangeably, depending on the types of problems they faced.

There are no rigid guidelines available on the best way to cope with stress. However, most researchers agree that no single coping mechanism is necessarily appropriate for dealing with all of life's stresses. They suggest that the more coping responses you can draw on, the better. Here are some coping techniques you can use for dealing with stress:

• *Exercise.* Almost any program of physical activity can help you overcome problems of stress. A regularly scheduled workout is excellent, if you can manage one, but even little things are helpful. Take a walk, play a game of tennis, weed the garden; activities like these are both physically and mentally good for you. (For more information on how exercise affects mental well-being, see Chapter ii).

• *Take time to relax.* Sometimes the best way to deal with stress is to get away from the stressful situation. Set aside a daily, quiet period for yourself. If you can, take a short nap. Otherwise schedule a ten- or fifteen-minute rest period at lunch or after work.

There are many useful relaxation techniques you can use to help combat stress. These techniques are often taught in short courses offered by local park districts, the YMCA and adult-education programs. The sessions are usually called stress-management or meditation courses. Check to see what is available in your community.

• *Develop new interests.* A stimulating avocation is one of the best antidotes to ordinary stress. If you have a hobby or outside interest, you can more easily escape the problems and tensions of daily life. Almost all of us have an old hobby we have ignored for years or an activity we have always wanted to pursue but never did. Now is a good time to develop these interests.

• *Seek advice.* The worst thing you can do is to keep your problems pent up inside. The best action is to talk about your concerns with others. Sharing your problems with friends, family members or religious advisors lets you get a better perspective and can provide new ideas on how to deal with them. If you feel overwhelmed by life's problems, you may need professional guidance. Ask your physician for advice.

• *Take positive action.* Once you identify the cause of your stress, whatever it might be, you should analyze the situation to see if there is anything you can do to correct or avoid the problem. If you are bothered by a relative's endless complaints, for example, talk to that person less often. If you are struggling to fit work, church, school and family activities and responsibilities into your schedule and find you cannot accomplish all of your goals, perhaps you need to face the fact that your ambitions are unrealistic. Rather than doing too much at once, set up a list of priorities, postpone some activities and take a slower, calmer approach to life.

• *Monitor personal habits.* Ask yourself if you are drinking too much, smoking too much, overeating or developing a dependency on drugs, such as sleeping aids or tranquilizers. If you are doing any or all of these things, it could mean you are under stress and are trying to relieve your tensions in an unhealthful fashion. Once you recognize this, you can take steps to correct it by substituting positive coping mechanisms, such as those just mentioned, for negative ones.

At the Baltimore (Maryland) Gerontology Research Center, scientists have found that attitude can play an important role in decreasing the amount of stress you encounter in life. Says Dr. Costa, you will experience less stress if you have a less rigid view toward life. If you feel you are entitled to certain rewards—no matter what they are—you will feel personally threatened if your life does not measure up to those expectations. For the sake of your health and mental well-being it is better to take the view that nothing is owed you and that everything in life is a challenge.

Problems of Depression

In the fourth century B.C., Hippocrates called the problem melancholia. In the twentieth century we know it as depression, a disorder that by conservative calculation affects between 5 and 20 percent of the population. According to medical estimates, one in every ten women and one in every twenty men will in their lifetimes endure depression severe enough to require medical treatment.

There are two periods during life in which adults seem particularly susceptible to the disease. The first is early adulthood, between the mid-twenties and the early thirties. The second is mid-life, specifically during the fifties.

Not all middle-aged adults will suffer from depression, but many will. Of patients forty-five to sixty-four years old who were admitted to state mental hospitals in one recent year, 12.3 percent were diagnosed as suffering from depression. In private psychiatric units, the figure was 55 percent. And we have no way of knowing how many others in that age group were treated by family doctors or private psychiatrists. The available data probably reflect only the tip of the iceberg.

No one knows for sure why the middle-aged are likely targets for depression. For years, menopause was thought to be a primary cause of depression in middle-aged women, but that notion has been disproved (see Chapter 7). Today, most experts agree that illness, physiological change associated with aging and life stresses may play a role in the development of the disorder. There are also indications that a tendency toward or susceptibility to depression may be an inherited trait. In other words, if there is a history of depression in your direct family line, you may be at an increased risk.

That is the bad news about depression. The good news is that depression is now better understood and more readily treatable than ever before in human history. Today medical science can counter depression with therapies unknown thirty years ago. Doctors can offer hope denied past victims of this often debilitating disorder.

Depression is recognized as a mood disorder that can affect both attitude and behavior. There are different types of depression. In some instances clear distinctions can be drawn between one form of depression and another but, in many cases, the boundaries blur and overlap.

Exogenous depression is defined as depression that arises from an external source. If it is *reactive depression,* it develops in response to a specific event or factor, such as stress or personal loss. If it is *toxic depression,* it generally represents an individual, adverse reaction to a prescribed medication. (Physicians usually treat this type of depression by either altering the dosage of the medication or substituting another appropriate drug in its place.)

But not all depression can be traced to specific causes. Some depressions are *endogenous.* They seem literally to spring from within, with no apparent external cause.

Just as the cause of depression can vary, so too can the intensity of the disorder. Severe depression that requires hospitalization or long-term, extensive treatment represents only a small percentage of the total number of cases treated. Most instances of depression are "mild depressions." Mild depression tends to be relatively short-lived and is usually highly responsive to short-term treatment.

Depression can affect anyone, so it is important that you be able to recognize its symptoms. These may vary slightly, depending on the exact nature of the problem, but in general, you should watch for the following signs:

• *Sleep disturbance.* Both sleeping too little and sleeping too much are common signs of depression. One person may be up half the night, another may sleep through half the day and both may be suffering from depression.

• *Loss of appetite.* Suddenly, you have no taste for food. Nothing appeals to you, not even a favorite dish, and no amount of coaxing can prompt you to eat properly. You begin avoiding meals. You cancel lunch dates or, worse, order a drink instead of a meal.

• *Fatigue.* You are suddenly tired all the time. You begin activities and cannot complete them. You are listless and lacking in energy.

• *Loss of interest in life.* If you are depressed, you have no desire to participate in the world around you. You don't care to read, you stop going to the theater, you let your sports tickets go unused.

• *An inability to concentrate.* Chances are, if you are suffering from depression, you pay little or no attention to the people and events around you. You may watch a television program and not be able to recall the story; you may listen to a conversation and not remember what was discussed.

• *Feelings of inferiority.* These can be expressed as self-deprecation ("I'm not good enough for this job") or mild paranoia ("They're out to get me; nobody likes me"). You lack confidence; you give up on a task because you know ahead of time you cannot succeed in completing it.

• *Sexual dysfunction.* Depression affects both sexual desire and the ability to perform (see Chapter 10 for details). Although the depressed person may feel that his or her sexual life is over, this is not true. Once the problem is treated, sexual activity usually returns to normal.

• *Behavioral and attitudinal changes.* Depression can temporarily alter the very nature of your character. A talkative person may become withdrawn; a shy individual, loudly gregarious. Any change in behavior that makes an individual "not like himself" may be a sign of depression.

It is critical to realize that you do not have to exhibit all of these symptoms to be depressed. Any one of these can be a sign of depression. If you recognize any of the symptoms in yourself, you may be suffering from the disease and should seek medical care.

Unfortunately, many depressed people are not aware that they are ill, or they find it easy to deny or to rationalize their situation. If you recognize signs of depression in close friends or family members, it is important that you talk to them and suggest a visit to their physician.

How can you distinguish depression from simple unhappiness? One sure sign is an inability to respond to positive events, says Jan Fawcett, M.D., director of the department of psychiatry at Rush-Presbyterian-St. Luke's Medical Center, Chicago, Illinois. At times we all experience unhappiness or a sense of feeling down. But we will react to positive circumstances when they occur. A severely depressed person will not. A depressed person will not feel better even if he or she wins a state lottery. Nor will the depressed individual express any optimism or sense of happiness if he is promoted, if his favorite team hits a winning streak or if any good fortune befalls him. To a depressed man or woman, none of this matters. Life is miserable anyway. Good fortune makes no difference. The person is turned off completely.

This is the insidious nature of depression. It robs its victims of self-esteem, confidence and optimism. It sentences them to a vicious, debilitating cycle of hopelessness that permeates their entire existence and often wreaks havoc on job performance, home life and social relationships. In short, depression can be "a living hell."

For years, the victims themselves were often blamed for their own depression. People were supposed to rise above their problems. If they could not, they were considered weak. That onus no longer exists. In the late 1950s, scientific evidence began to indicate that, at least in some instances, biochemical imbalances in the body can generate depression. These data have been largely substantiated, although the underlying question of which comes first, the chicken or the egg, remains unresolved. For example, do psychological pressures cause chemical changes responsible for depression? Or do chemical changes result in a state that undermines the victim's ability to cope with life's stresses?

Although the exact mechanics of depression remain unclear, effective treatments have been developed. Depression therapies are psychological, chemical and electrical in nature. They may be used singularly or in some combination, depending upon the patient and the severity of the disorder. In some instances, changes in life-style and increased physical activity (see Chapter 11) also are effective in helping combat depression.

Psychological therapy involves various forms of verbal communication, in which a professional therapist attempts to improve the patient's capacity to cope. Psychological therapy is generally very successful in treating mild forms of depression.

One of the newest and most promising of the verbal techniques is an approach known as cognitive therapy, developed by Aaron T. Beck, M.D., professor of psychiatry at the University of Pennsylvania School of Medicine and director of the Mood Clinic at the University Hospital, Philadelphia. Cognitive therapy is based on the premise that depression has its roots in a negative view of the self, the world and the future. Moods do not influence thought as we have traditionally believed, says Dr. Beck. Rather, thoughts influence moods. To fight depression, cognitive therapists teach people to recognize and challenge what are found to be consistently negative thought patterns.

"We are not creating Pollyannas or preaching positive thinking," explains Arthur Freeman, Ph.D., of the Center for Cognitive Therapy at the University of Pennsylvania. "We want to help the depressed person divide his life processes into workable problems. Then we target in on these one by one. We show the person that no matter what the difficulty is, he has choices." The cognitive-therapy process, says Dr. Freeman, is essentially the same for the middle-aged man who is depressed because he has lost his job or because his son is involved with drugs as it is for the fifty-five-year-old professional who, although successful by society's standards, is depressed because she feels she has not measured up to her own standards. In each instance, the patient is helped to focus on reality and to identify steps he or she can take to improve the situation.

How successful is cognitive therapy in combating depression? In one study of forty-one severely depressed patients, some 78 percent showed complete remission or marked improvement. In general, other studies also attest to the effectiveness of the therapy.

Another mode of treatment for depression is found in the new psychopharmacology. This form of treatment is based on chemical or drug therapy. Prior to the 1950s, effective drug therapy for depression was not available. Today, there are three medications that can be used: lithium (for cyclic episodes of manic depression) and tricyclics and monamine oxidase inhibitors (the antidepressives). The antidepressives, of which there are many, affect the brain's functioning by stimulating the activity of neurotransmitters (chemicals that transmit impulses from one brain cell to another).

Psychopharmacology does have drawbacks, however. First, antidepressive drugs require a certain amount of time, once taken, to be effective; a few days or several weeks may elapse between treatment initiation and patient response. Second, the drugs may produce side effects, including a dry mouth, blurry vision and tremors. "The side effects are not usually medically serious," says Rush-Presbyterian-St. Luke's Dr. Fawcett, "but to the depressed patient who is already discouraged and convinced that nothing will help, they represent another burden." Third, drug effectiveness varies with each patient and with the dosage taken. Too much of an antidepressive drug can be as ineffective as too little. A drug that produces a complete reversal of symptoms in one patient may be ineffective in another.

Until recently there was little information available to guide physicians in matching medication and dosage to specific patients. Today that is changing. "We can now measure drug levels in the blood," says Dr. Fawcett. "And we are developing ways of predicting in advance which medication to use first. For example, we can give a patient a challenged dose of a stimulant drug. If that patient responds to the stimulant, then we know to which antidepressive drug he will also respond."

A third method of treatment is electroshock therapy (EST). Like drug therapy, EST stimulates the production of neurotransmitters, but does so using, as the stimulus, electricity, not chemicals. EST is generally reserved for very severe cases of depression. In its present form it is considered a procedure that is safe and appropriate for most adults. Memory loss is a common side effect, but the problem is usually temporary.

Depression is a highly complex problem. It may appear in cycles. It may present itself as a once-in-a-lifetime event. It can persist for long periods, "masked" or hidden behind a general sense of listlessness, disinterest and despair. Severe depression can result, in some instances, in suicide. Left untreated, depression can disappear on its own, perhaps after months or years of haunting its victim.

"Depression is so common that people often consider it one of life's cruelties rather than an illness," says Dr. Fawcett. "They view it as a condition of unhappiness that is warranted by some life event and not as a treatable medical problem."

For people in their fifties, depression poses a particular threat because many of the changes that depression induces can easily be confused with the stereotypical behavior society equates with aging. In some instances, depressed middle-aged adults have no idea they are suffering from a medical illness because their symptoms match behavior that society says means they are growing older. They dismiss their disinterest, fatigue and withdrawal as being normal "for their age."

There is no reason for people to feel that way, says Dr. Fawcett. We attribute certain characteristics—joy of life, optimism and high expectations for the future—to youth, but these are human characteristics. They belong to the middle-aged as well.

7

UNDERSTANDING THE FEMALE MENOPAUSE AND THE MALE CLIMACTERIC

When women get together to talk about menopause, they say things like the following:

• "My periods became irregular last year, and for the first time now I missed two in a row. A few months ago I started having hot flashes, but they fluctuate. I think I'm in the beginning stages of menopause, but I don't really know."

• "My mother started menopause when she was thirty, and even as a child I was aware of her discomfort. She was really miserable. I decided to be as natural about bodily functions as I could. I was going to take my menopause as smoothly as possible. But when it came, a lot of other things were happening. I didn't have a regular doctor, one who knew my history, and I developed a breast cyst and didn't know what was going on. I was on an emotional whirlwind and I don't know if it was related to menopause or not."

• "The lack of information on menopause and the bodily changes that occur are so vast, I was angry when I began to experience it. I went for information and found very little. People were very cavalier, and I felt like I was supposed to ignore everything that was happening to me."

The conversation continued for nearly two hours as the women in a discussion group sponsored by the Consumers Health Center in Evanston, Illinois, shared their experiences and ideas about menopause. This was the first time the women had met; yet they exhibited no hesitancy in their willingness to talk. They listened attentively as one woman described the increased level of flow she experienced just before she began skipping periods. They laughed sympathetically as another related her husband's reaction to a menopausal night sweat. "He turned over to me and went, 'Yech,' and I was so hurt—he hasn't done that again."

They broached the subject of changing sexual needs and of the sense of loneliness that, to date, has permeated so much of the menopausal experience. These women were searching for specific information on symptoms as well as for the elusive sense of relief that comes when unspoken fears are finally revealed. As the women talked, it became clear that to them menopause means more than simply cessation of periods for a twelve-month span. They view it in a very real sense as a rite of passage from one stage of life to another; they experience it as an event with important implications that can influence almost every aspect of their lives.

In the past, many roadblocks have been constructed in the menopausal maze. Most of these are simply old tales. They evolved from misconception and misinformation and are being refuted with fact and modern research. To understand the menopause it is important to realize that throughout history, almost all aspects of menopause have been influenced by society's views toward women and the female climacteric. For a look at how ideas and attitudes have evolved through time, see page 77, "Menopause: A Historical Perspective."

Recently, the Society for Menstrual Cycle Research, headquartered in Chicago, sponsored an international symposium on menopause at the University of Arizona, Tucson. The overriding message was highly positive. The theme that ran through all presentations at the conference was the same theme that circled the table of women gathered that one afternoon: Women can cope with menopause. "The essence was that we can move through anything we understand and handle it quite effectively," says Ann M. Voda, Ph.D., director of the Physiological Nursing Program at the University of Utah School of Nursing, Salt Lake City, and coordinator of the meeting. "It's just that, not too long ago, nothing was known except the old wive's tales that have been perpetuated."

Following are some of the most common myths that we hear about menopause and the facts that refute them.

Myth 1. Menopause is medically defined as a disease.

Not true—at least not anymore. For years many doctors and lay people thought of menopause as an illness, a condition requiring medical treatment, but that attitude has since changed. What menopause *is* is a deficiency syndrome, in that the secretion of estrogen is diminished. As a consequence, some degenerative changes may occur, such as osteoporosis (a loss of bone density), which may or may not require medical attention. (Osteoporosis is discussed in detail later in this chapter.)

But oftentimes what happens is that doctors see only those women having problems, and this colors their view of the menopausal experience, explains Mary Jane Gray, M.D., adjunct professor of obstetrics and gynecology at the University of North Carolina Medical School, Chapel Hill. If the only women who mention menopause are those having troubles, the doctor develops the view that all women have problems. In reality, though, the majority are quietly going about their lives, are not having problems and are *not* discussing it with their physicians. As more women began talking about their experiences with menopause, as they began reassessing the event in different terms, the emphasis shifted, says Dr. Gray. "Today menopause is not considered an illness; rather it is accepted as a normal, developmental phase in a woman's life, and I think everyone feels that this whole re-evaluation is a healthy one."

Most women experience menopause between the ages of forty-five and fifty-five. In most instances, the menopausal transition period takes two to three years to complete, although in some cases the process may last anywhere from ten to fifteen years. Some women notice definite physical changes, such as an unusual degree of breast sensitivity, a tendency to retain water or a stiffening of the finger joints, long before their periods become irregular. But for many, skipped periods and fluctuations between unusually light and heavy flow are the first indications that menopause is beginning.

Medically, a woman is considered premenopausal up to the time her periods cease for a full twelve months. She is menopausal only during that one year and is postmenopausal from that time on. No woman really knows for sure where she stands until that decisive twelve-month span has already been completed. That is the cutoff point, after which a woman usually cannot become pregnant. Until a woman is definitely postmenopausal, she should continue using birth control devices.

The physiological changes of menopause might seem simple, but they are so interdependent that the end result is a highly complex process. It is just not enough to say that "the ovaries stop functioning." Menopause means more than that, because the ovaries do not operate in a vacuum.

During a woman's active reproductive life, the ovaries are set in motion every month by a chain reaction of events that involves part of the brain called the hypothalamus, the pituitary gland, and two gonadotropic hormones—the follicle-stimulating hormone (FSH) and the luteinizing hormone (LH). With the right orchestration from the hypothalamus and the pituitary, FSH and LH descend on the ovary and switch it into action. Basically, the ovary has two tasks. It matures egg cells for potential release into the uterus and it secretes estrogen, which stimulates tissue growth on the wall of the uterus—in preparation for implantation of a fertilized egg. At the proper time a burst of LH is sent to the ovaries, triggering the ovulation of one, rarely two, selected ova. If a woman becomes pregnant, the cycle stops; if not, it continues. The ovarian follicles halt the flow of estrogen and begin producing progesterone, the hormone that sloughs off the extra tissue built up in the uterus. This results in menstrual flow.

Menopause brings an end to all this activity, and the ovaries, pituitary and hypothalamus must now come into a new, harmonious balance that will continue throughout the postmenopausal stage. The winding-down period is not always smooth. Body signals can be misread; timing may be off as one organ or another awaits the proper hormonal signal to begin or cease its activity; the pituitary may produce incredibly large amounts of FSH and LH to try to keep the ovaries functioning as before; and periods become irregular.

Eventually, periods cease altogether, and the body, having reached a different plateau of operation, continues in its new state of equilibrium.

The range of individual biological differences in response to menopause is enormous, making it virtually impossible to describe a "normal" or "typical" experience. Hot flashes, including "night sweats," may occur in some women. They tend to taper off as the physiological adjustment to the menopause is completed, but can endure for years. Vaginal atrophy, a thinning and drying out of the vaginal wall associated with decreased estrogen levels, may also be present and may extend into the postmenopausal years, often causing dyspareunia, or pain during intercourse. While it is safe to say that most women are affected by menopausal symptoms, the degree to which they are bothered and the question of whether or not medical treatment is indicated are bound up in more of the myths surrounding the phenomenon.

Myth 2. After menopause, women no longer produce natural estrogen and need full replacement of this hormone.

Although the ovaries stop manufacturing estrogen, the postmenopausal woman is not completely lacking the hormone from other body sources. In fact, there are two such natural sources. Estrogens come directly from the adrenal cortex, part of the adrenal gland, which literally sits on top of the kidneys, and indirectly from the body's adipose tissue, or fat cells, which converts androgens to estrogen. Ironically, the ovaries, which no longer secrete estrogen, continue to produce small amounts of androgens, which eventually wind up as estrogens.

However, neither of these alternative sources produces as much of or the same type of estrogen—there are three kinds (estrone, estradiol and estriol)—as the functioning ovaries do in the premenopausal woman. "There is clearly a deficiency of estrogen in the postmenopausal woman in the sense that the level of estrogens drops from the time she is menstruating to the time she is menopausal," explains Mortimer B. Lipsett, M.D., of the National Institutes of Health in Bethesda, Maryland. "But the real question is whether the deficiency *needs* to be replaced." According to Dr. Lipsett, medical science is still accumulating the data that will one day provide the definitive answer (see page 80 in this chapter for a discussion of the pros and cons of estrogen-replacement therapy).

Meanwhile another question remains foremost in the minds of

many middle-aged women: Is estrogen therapy safe? The answer depends, in large part, on whether you are talking about short-term or long-term estrogen-replacement therapy (ERT). Short-term use generally involves treatment of menopausal symptoms and is accepted as both safe and appropriate. Long-term use today is considered both controversial and appropriate only for countering bone loss in women, a problem discussed later in this chapter.

In 1975, the first two of seven reports were published that linked ERT to endometrial cancer, or cancer of the uterine wall. Among menopausal and postmenopausal women who do not use estrogen and who have their uteri intact, endometrial cancer occurs in approximately one tenth of 1 percent of the population. When detected early, usually through irregular bleeding, the cancer can be successfully treated by hysterectomy.

According to a four-year study of some 1,300 patients at six hospitals in the Baltimore, Maryland, area, women using estrogen for more than five years have a fifteen times greater chance of developing endometrial cancer than nonusers. The Boston (Massachusetts) Collaborative Drug Surveillance Program of Boston University Medical Center says the risk is from ten to thirty times greater. To date, however, estrogen has not been associated with cancer in short-term users, those who might take the drug for less than two years; and, according to the Boston research, the risk of developing endometrial cancer reverses once the drug is no longer taken.

Both the American Council on Science and Health and the National Institutes of Health Consensus Development Conference on Estrogen Use and Postmenopausal Women agree that women should not take estrogen to slow the aging process, increase sensuality, counter psychological disorders or protect against heart disease; it doesn't work for these purposes. But estrogen remains the only recognized effective treatment available for hot flashes and, in certain cases, dyspareunia.

"If a woman has severe hot flashes, everyone agrees she should take estrogen for that period—sometimes for six months or one year, rarely for two years," says Dr. Lipsett, president of the Endocrine Society. "If a woman has dyspareunia and has trouble with intercourse as a result, then estrogen certainly is indicated, but the length of time to give it depends on an assessment of the other risks and benefits. If a woman says, 'I don't need estrogen; I'm active and am having no hot flashes or problems,' you wouldn't argue with her."

For some women, estrogen is definitely contraindicated or inadvisable. These include women who have had breast cancer; those who suffer from severe migraine headaches, which the hormone can exacerbate; and those with a history of fibroid tumors or high blood pressure. Some self-help books suggest taking vitamin E for treating both hot flashes and dyspareunia, and there are a few existing medical reports supporting its effectiveness with these symptoms. But the recommended doses are often very high, can cause stomach and intestinal discomfort or blurred vision and are contraindicated for women with high blood pressure, diabetes or rheumatic heart condition.

Myth 3. Depression and mental instability are a natural part of menopause.

In 1857, British physician Dr. Edward J. Tilt wrote that "a large class of women are thoroughly unhinged by the change of life . . . eccentricity embitters their existence and . . . the nervous symptoms of the change of life assume vast importance." Dr. Tilt was referring to a phenomenon known as involutional melancholia, or the menopausal syndrome. Symptoms were wide ranging, and included anxiety, depression, irritability, emotional instability, headache, insomnia, fatigue and apathy. Both society and medicine attributed the syndrome to the "raging" hormonal imbalances of menopause and nodded sympathetically whenever a woman approached the "change." She would take her chances in a world that had stacked the odds against her. She could become neurotic, warned Sigmund Freud; she would suffer "partial death," said psychoanalyst Helene Deutsch. Even as recently as the 1960s, menopause was associated with the dismal prospect of becoming a eunuch or of existing in "living decay."

In fact, there is little proof linking psychiatric illness to menopause. Clinical depression is no more prevalent among menopausal women than among women of other ages and, as for Dr. Tilt's involutional melancholia, only about six out of every 100,000 menopausal women are victims of the disorder. At best, some of the symptoms attributed to menopause are really spin-offs of other stresses that develop during mid-life or that may be only indirectly related to the change of life itself. A woman who loses sleep from hot flashes might well be irritable, not because of menopause but because of a lack of proper rest. A benchmark study headed by human development expert Bernice L. Neugarten, Ph.D., further showed that the alleged "psychological" symptoms of menopause affect women across the board and are most frequently encountered by *adolescents,* not by menopausal women. In another survey of pre- and post-menopausal women, Dr. Neugarten found that the anticipation of menopause was worse than the actual experience of it. The women with the most negative ideas and attitudes were women who had not yet gone through that stage of life.

The women who might have the most difficulty with menopause are those who most highly value motherhood. Even they can make a successful transition, however. What's important are the kind of options women have available.

Myth 4. Almost all menopausal women suffer from severe and incapacitating hot flashes.

The actual figure is closer to 10 percent, meaning that the great majority of women are not victimized by the hot flash or flush.

In a preliminary study of 115 women, Dr. Voda identified three types of hot-flash symptoms: mild, moderate and severe. Mild hot flashes ended in less than one minute, involved little noticeable perspiration and did not interfere with normal activity. Moderate symptoms made the individual slightly uncomfortable (to the point where she might remove a layer of clothing), involved noticeable perspiration and lasted more than one minute. Severe flashes were characterized by marked sweating, lasted for more than two minutes and forced the subject to interrupt her normal activity. "A woman can have all three kinds of hot flashes," says Dr. Voda. "But it's the severe one that doesn't show up very often. In this study, fewer women had severe symptoms than had either mild or moderate."

The hot flash is linked to changes in the diameter of the blood vessels, but scientists are not sure what causes the changes or exactly how they occur. Now researchers at the University of California, San Diego, indicate that the entire process may be more complex than previously thought. They implicate a physiological chain of events similar to that involved in the menstrual cycle. This would include estrogen as well as the gonadotropic hormones (follicle-stimulating hormone and luteinizing hormone) and certain brain neurons.

When a woman has a hot flash, she becomes warm, often perspires and may sense a reddening in the face. (Although internal body temperature falls following a hot flash, skin temperature tends to rise, in some instances as much as seven or more degrees.) Then the heat is gone, and she becomes chilled.

Dr. Gray, of the University of North Carolina School of Medicine, says that, although some women are embarrassed by hot flashes, in general a hot flash is not as obvious as one might think. "It looks like a blush," she explains. "If someone were really paying attention, he or she might notice, but no one really does. It's rare that people go around labeling women as having hot flashes."

In the next phase of her work, Dr. Voda plans to compare women with hot flashes and women without them to determine if body type and the percentage of body fat make any difference. Theoretically, women with more adipose tissue synthesize more estrogen than thin women and should not have the same experience with hot flashes. The theory remains to be proved, but so far Dr. Voda's research has revealed two consistent patterns in the hot-flash experience.

First, each of the 115 volunteers in the study had a specific focal point where the heat sensation inevitably began. This ranged from top of the head, to the cheekbones, the area between the breasts and, for one woman, the left ear. This does not mean, however, that the focal point is always so specific. Some women, in fact, consistently perceived the heat sensation all over (total body perception). Second, for each subject, the hot-flash spread was very predictable and seemed to follow a particular pattern. While for some the flash remained an upper-body phenomenon, for others the patterns involved portions of the pelvis and the legs as well as the upper torso (see diagrams, pages 72-73).

Data from the study indicate that hot flashes tend to occur more often at night than during the day. They seem less tied to stress than to sleep-related activities. Finally, says Dr. Voda, the research shows that most women, even those with severe symptoms, cope well with hot flashes. "When you match the myth against the reality, it's the fear and the tales that cause the most anxiety."

Myth 5. A woman who has had a hysterectomy will not experience natural menopause in mid-life.

This depends on the extent of the surgery. When physicians refer to *partial hysterectomy*, they mean removal of the uterus only; when they use the term *total hysterectomy*, they mean removal of the uterus and the cervix, and sometimes the ovaries. Only a bilateral oophorectomy, or removal of both ovaries, will produce a surgically imposed menopause, and whereas by age fifty approximately 30 percent of women have had hysterectomies, less than half have also had a bilateral oophorectomy. If a woman has either one or both ovaries remaining after a hysterectomy, she will still experience a natural menopause during mid-life as her ovarian function winds down. To avoid confusion, a woman undergoing a hysterectomy should make sure she clearly understands the extent of the surgery to be performed.

Myth 6. Sexual desire ends with menopause.

In the past, society has assumed that older women are not sexually active. In many instances, men thought their wives' menopausal experience meant the end of their sexual relationship. In more recent times, these views have been proved invalid. The reality for many women is that by the time they reach menopause they find themselves enjoying sex more than when they were worried about birth control and pregnancy. Often, in fact, the women are more interested in sex than the men. One study at Duke University, Durham, North Carolina, has found that among many middle-aged couples, husbands, not wives, were typically the ones responsible for halting sexual relations.

More recently, the Boston (Massachusetts) Women's Collective distributed 2,000 questionnaires on menopause to women across the country. One question asked women if they felt different about

The Hot Flash Experience

The hot flash, or hot flush, as it is commonly referred to, is the result of complex physiological changes that occur in the body, in some women, during menopause and, not infrequently, in the post menopausal years.

Recent studies conducted by Ann M. Voda, Ph.D., of the University of Minnesota School of Nursing, have shown that no two women who experience hot flashes will have the same symptoms. That is, the degree of intensity of the hot flash and the spread of the flush on the body will differ from woman to woman.

Below are actual case histories taken from the Voda study which illustrate common types of hot flash symptoms experienced by women in their fifties.

---

1. Perceived origin and spread of the hot flash for a 57 year-old housewife experiencing natural menopause who recorded 21 hot flashes over a two-week

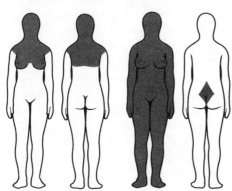

period. Seventeen hot flashes originated in the "neck to breast" area while four originated in the "neck up and breast" area, including the back and shoulders. Regardless of the point of origin the subject described the hot flash spread as encompassing the entire front of the body but restricted to the sacroiliac area of the back.

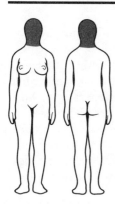

2. A 56 year-old woman experiencing natural menopause recorded 35 hot flashes over a two-week period. All 35 hot flashes originated in the same area encompassing the entire neck and head. The downward spread of the hot flash encompassed the front and back of the body and remained an upper body phenomenon.

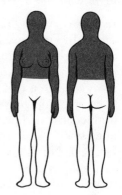

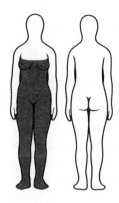

3. Perceived origin and spread of the hot flash for a 58 year-old woman who recorded 114 hot flashes over a two-week period. Origin of the hot flash was confined to "breasts and below." Ninety-five hot flashes spread "up" from the point of origin while 19 spread "all over" frontally.

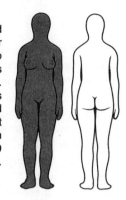

4. A 59 year-old housewife experiencing natural menopause recorded 27 hot flashes over a two-week period. All hot flashes originated in the "neck and up" area, specifically the face and back of the head and excluding the top of the head. All of the hot flashes spread "down," excluding the top of the head, the arms below the elbow, the hands, both feet and the posterior lower legs.

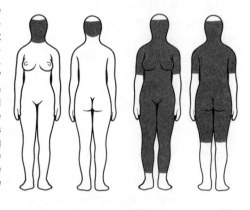

Source: Ann M. Voda, Ph.D., University of Minnesota School of Nursing

themselves sexually. Two thirds of the menopausal and post-menopausal women who responded said no. In addition, half reported no change in sexual desire, while about 25 percent noted an increase. However, 25 percent reported a decrease in desire.

For some women, this lack of interest in sex presents no dilemma and may even be welcome. For others, the shift can be traumatic. "I mourn for the person I used to be," explained one woman in the menopause discussion group cited earlier. "It's not that I suddenly dislike sex, I simply have no interest any longer, and this bothers me."

Traditionally, a drop in sexual interest in the menopausal woman was associated with a decrease in estrogen, but this thinking is being challenged. There are indications that it is the hormone androgen, not estrogen, that plays a significant role in female sexual desire. Although androgen is a male hormone, it is also present in small amounts in women, and, like estrogen, it decreases during the menopause. While some women will lose their sexual interest purely on psychological grounds, research indicates that for others the problem could be linked to a reduction in androgens. Additional research is needed, however, before scientists will know to what extent the decrease in sexual desire is linked to biogenic causes, and how these might be treated.

Some women suffer from vaginal atrophy, a thinning and drying of the vaginal wall associated with decreased estrogen levels. Although this can cause dyspareunia, or painful intercourse, some women claim that sexual activity itself is an effective antidote and that abstinence only makes the problem worse. Dyspareunia can be treated with estrogen, taken either orally in pill form or applied locally in cream form. The Consensus Conference—a National Institutes of Health meeting—cautions that estrogens in vaginal creams may be absorbed quickly into the bloodstream and has called for more research into their long-term effects. Women who use the creams should remain under the supervision of their physician.

Myth 7. There is no life after menopause.

The late anthropologist Margaret Mead, Ph.D., noted that women were often peppier after menopause than they had been before. She called the phenomenon PMZ—postmenopausal zest. In Dr.

Neugarten's study of women's attitudes toward menopause, two women talked about their experiences in the postmenopausal period. "I've been healthier and in much better spirits since 'the change of life,' " said one. "Since I've had my menopause, I have felt like a teenager again," reported another. "I can remember my mother saying that after her menopause she really got her vigor, and I can say the same thing about myself. I'm just never tired now."

Researchers suggest that a number of factors can account for the existence of postmenopausal zest. For one thing, postmenopausal women no longer have to contend with the occasional mild anemia they may have experienced because of menstrual periods. For another, women are freed from the mood swings that, for some, characterized their monthly cycles. After menopause, women also no longer have to worry about birth control techniques and possible late-life pregnancies. Those who have reared children are, by this time, freed from many of their earlier familial responsibilities. For many women, these changes can have a positive psychological effect on their attitudes toward life.

Myth 8. Men are not affected by a woman's menopause.

Until recently, no one has really bothered to ask them. Research on the subject in this country comes from two undergraduate women at Michigan State University, East Lansing, who recently completed a nine-family pilot study they hope will set the stage for further investigation into menopause from the family's perspective.

In their survey, Jacqueline Gretzinger and Kristi Dege went beyond the traditional scope of the menopausal experience. They returned with a blurred and largely negative picture of menopause, one drawn by an uncertain and often confused audience made up of teenage children and husbands.

In a sense the researchers were lucky to get any picture at all. "We don't talk about it," was the most common response the women heard as they searched for families willing to participate in the study. One after another, their inquiries were shunted aside until, finally, after three months of searching, they had their subjects in hand.

"We found that family members were concerned about the wife

and mother and wanted to make life easier for her during this
period," explains Gretzinger. "But at the same time we learned
that children know virtually nothing about menopause and that
men know very little. They get most of their information from the
media—newspapers, magazines and television. In fact, a number
of participants said they learned about menopause by sharing
Edith Bunker's experience on an episode of the television series
All in the Family."

For the most part, men maintain the basic attitude that, until
recently, permeated the public and even professional view of menopause: No matter what happens to a woman at this time of life,
menopause is the culprit.

The biggest misconception Gretzinger and Dege discovered
was that menopause makes women "irritable and grouchy."
Men acknowledged that there were other pressures and other
changes going on at the time, such as children leaving home, but
they made no connection between these events and their wives'
behavior. A menopausal woman was irritable and grouchy,
and it was menopause alone that made women irritable and
grouchy.

One man in particular was disturbed because his wife had
become more assertive and independent. She balked at attending the church of his choice and was no longer the "yes, dear;
no, dear" spouse he had known all their married life. Worse yet,
he couldn't raise his voice at her anymore because "she'd
yell back." The entire problem, as he viewed it, was menopause.

Every man in the study had at least one answer when asked to
describe the "worst thing" about menopause. When asked what
the "best thing" was, half had no answer to give. The beliefs about
menopause the men expressed most frequently reflect their negative view:

- A woman is not the same person after menopause.
- Most women get depressed about the change of life.
- Women worry about going crazy during menopause.
- Life becomes less interesting for a woman after menopause.
- Menopause is an unpleasant experience, a disturbing event
  that most women dread.

While the men, all of whom were married and living with their spouses, felt they discussed menopause with and were more understanding of their wives during this period, some also admitted they weren't sure whether their wives were menopausal. In some instances, in fact, men identified their wives as menopausal when the women said they were not, or described their wives as not menopausal when the women said they were definitely in the menopause.

"The men weren't really sure if menopause was a disease or a normal process," says Gretzinger. "They knew nothing about postmenopause, and only those with more education thought of menopause in terms of actual physical changes. Still, it's refreshing that they disagreed with one of the major, old myths—that after menopause women don't consider themselves 'real women' anymore."

The bottom line in the Michigan study lays the burden for change on the woman in the family. Since she is the person experiencing menopause, say the researchers, it is her responsibility to communicate her feelings to other members of the family. They, in turn, must respond to her in a positive, supportive fashion and keep the lines of communication open.

MENOPAUSE: A HISTORICAL PERSPECTIVE

Throughout past generations, popular notions about menopause have been largely negative. Historically, however, menopause had been considered a beneficial event, and today it is again being viewed in a more positive light. In this special section, Anne M. Seiden, M.D., a nationally acknowledged expert on the psychology of women, explains why attitudes toward menopause have changed so drastically throughout human history. Dr. Seiden is director of the department of psychiatry at Cook County Hospital in Chicago. The following are her views on menopause:

Menopause is nature's original contraceptive. It guarantees that the average woman who reaches menopausal age will have many years of health and vigor after the birth of her last child. In the past, if a woman continued to have children until she died, she would be too busy with the care of small children to spend time transmitting to others what she had learned about child care and human nature. This is important. Human child rearing is not predominantly instinctive. We have to get it mostly from our culture, as did our ancestors. Although women in the past oftentimes died young, menopause ensured that tribes, for example, had a substantial number of older women who were not preoccupied with day-to-day care of small infants and who were therefore free to take a leadership role in the tribe. This phenomenon is unusual in the mammalian kingdom; of all mammals, possibly only rhesus monkeys share anything like this with us. All mammals have mother-infant relationships, but only humans have something like the grandmother-mother-infant triad. Only humans have "elders," half of whom are women, to provide cultural wisdom and leadership. Menopause probably makes possible a great deal of human culture as we know it.

When society became more complex, attitudes about menopause began to change. Menopause became linked with female sexuality, and female sexuality was often defined by men, not by women. In many patriarchal cultures, the most visible value of a woman was in bearing children. Wealthy men might have many wives, like they had many cattle. Children were economically valuable and were proof of their father's masculinity. From the man's perspective, a woman who ended her childbearing function might well be an obsolete animal—unless she were his favorite wife.

In this country alone we have been through several stages in our cultural history of menopause. When people were pioneers and living off the land, they were eager to have children. And, when menopause came, many women were glad to reach it—they'd had enough. There were no reliable contraceptives, except abstinence. Thus, menopause was not an unwelcome time for a large number of women. We also have to keep in mind that experiencing some of the symptoms associated with menopause, such as hot ashes, would certainly seem a small price to pay for the freedom from having any more children when you have already had all the children you want and there is no other way to be sure of preventing more pregnancies.

On the other hand, if there are other methods of contraception available in the culture, then the *onset* of menopause begins to lose some of its attraction. We begin to focus too much attention on symptoms only, and we forget what the symptoms are heralding—menopause and all of the positive meanings associated with it.

As indicated earlier, many women naturally moved into leadership roles after menopause. However, if a society holds women back from moving into such roles—if a woman has no productive outlet for her abilities—then tension and depression can result. For example, let us suppose that you are doing the same old housework, which actually never did seem very glamorous. But it seemed worthwhile when it was tied to the important task of rearing children. Then the anchor for that task is lifted—the children grow up. You are faced either with moving on to something else or left with a feeling of the beginning of the end. You visualize yourself carrying out the same old deadly routine, but no longer for any kind of ennobling purpose. At the same time, menopause comes to be defined as a disease. All these things happened together historically, and, as a consequence, in our society, menopause became a negative experience for many women.

Today we are again beginning to view menopause in a more positive light. And I think we are doing so because our culture looks more favorably upon women and also because women are doing more of the thinking and writing about menopause. In fact, many of the women who are thinking and writing about everything in our society are post-menopausal. They are our proof, our models. They are able to say, "No, the negative things associated with menopause are not true."

Of course, it is possible to experience sadness at menopause. The sadness can be very real for the woman who dreamed of having more children than she actually did—or who has other reasons for nostalgia about her early years. But who ever fulfills all of his or her early dreams, and who doesn't sometimes experience nostalgia? These are emotions associated with maturity—not just with menopause.

On the other hand, many women enjoy a sense of relief and achievement at menopause. For some, menopause is the beginning of genuine adult life. This is a feeling that more and more mature women are enjoying today.

Osteoporosis: More on the Estrogen Controversy

In the late 1930s, Fuller Albright, M.D., a physician at Massachusetts General Hospital, Boston, first linked menopause and a decrease in ovarian function to a marked increase in bone fractures
in older women. Scientists had known for years that aging women
were more likely than men to break their wrists, hipbones and
vertebrae, but generally attributed the problems to women being
the weaker sex or to the fact that—at least until the early part of
this century—they tripped over the long skirts that fashion dictated as their costume. Dr. Albright said no; women were particularly susceptible targets for osteoporosis, a condition best described as loss of bone mass. The physician-scientist argued that
estrogen helps bind calcium to bone and that a menopausal decrease in the level of estrogen in the body results in a loss of
calcium and thus a loss of bone. Lifelong estrogen replacement
therapy (ERT) would solve the problem, said Dr. Albright, who
was among the first to prescribe this treatment for women. Today,
Dr. Albright's theory is at the center of a spirited controversy not
only about the actual mechanics of the disease but also about the
recommended therapies, especially the use of estrogen. Although
its exact prevalence has not been established, it is thought that
about 25 percent of all postmenopausal women will develop clinical osteoporosis. Millions of women will suffer broken wrists, hip
fractures and the telltale collapsed vertebrae that lead to the loss
of height and the hunched shoulders seen so often in the elderly.
  Although we think of bone as a stable, nonchanging substance,
it is really in almost constant transition as calcium is deposited and
reabsorbed by the body. During childhood and adolescence, more
new bone is formed than old bone is dismantled. At some point
after the growth spurt ends, the amount of new bone being formed
equals the amount reabsorbed. This balance lasts until about age
twenty-five or thirty, when the equilibrium shifts. From then on,
more bone is broken down than is produced. The complications
of bone loss do not present as great a problem for men as they do
for women because men have more bone mass. They will lose
about 3 percent every decade, but they rarely develop the problems
of osteoporosis until possibly during advanced old age. For
women, the story is different. Starting in their mid to late thirties,

they lose about 8 percent of bone every decade, and for some, at menopause, the rate increases substantially. Women have less bone mass to begin with, so their loss is more critical. The only exceptions are black women, who, like men, start with denser bones, and even though they also lose bone mass, do not suffer the fractures of osteoporosis in later life.

Most research continues to support Dr. Albright's theories linking estrogen to bone loss, but other factors have also been implicated. Louis V. Avioli, M.D., has spent nearly two decades studying osteoporosis. Dr. Avioli, professor of medicine at Washington University, Saint Louis, Missouri, explains that bone loss can be aggravated by a sedentary life-style, improper balance of phosphorus and calcium in the diet, diabetes, smoking and excessive alcohol consumption. Changes in the intestinal tract as one ages often result in decreased calcium absorption in the body, and subtle metabolic alterations governed by the thyroid and parathyroid glands can add to the complications. Sometimes, changes in bone result not from osteoporosis but from another, similar condition called osteomalacia. Osteoporosis affects bone quantity, not bone quality. Osteomalacia, on the other hand, may or may not alter quantity, but always affects the quality of the bone and should be treated first. The only way to distinguish between the two conditions is through a bone biopsy, a simple and painless procedure performed with a local anesthetic.

Until recently, scientists had few early warning signs for osteoporosis itself. Localized back pain, one symptom, is rare. Most X rays cannot detect the condition until some 40 to 50 percent of bone is already lost. Even laboratory tests prove ineffectual because, ironically, women with osteoporosis have the same levels of circulating estrogen in their bodies as women without the disease.

But as researchers unravel the complexities of osteoporosis, they also discover new ways of detecting and treating the disease. A simple film or X ray of the hand may now provide the key to early diagnosis. It is effective in measuring subtle telltale osteoporotic changes in the metacarpal (hand) bones and should soon become more widely used.

Recommendations for therapy range from dietary changes and calcium supplements to vitamin D treatment, especially for those with osteomalacia (softening of the bone). Experimental techniques are also being tested. These include supplements of sodium fluoride to stimulate bone formation, and calcitonin, a hormone from the thyroid gland, to suppress bone reabsorption. Today an established and controversial treatment is estrogen replacement therapy (ERT). The question is, Who should be put on ERT and for how long?

Critics claim that no definitive X-ray proof has ever been presented to show that estrogen itself prevents bone loss and reduces risk of fracture. They argue that short-term estrogen therapy is helpful but that long-term treatment may actually contribute to accelerated bone loss. Complications of estrogen therapy, such as gallbladder disease, high blood pressure, strokes and breast cancer in patients with a family history of such, also must be considered. Finally, the risk of cancer is too great, according to the opponents of ERT, to warrant the therapy for all menopausal women. Those who defend estrogen therapy claim that X-ray proof of bone formation is no criterion for measuring the efficacy of estrogen in halting bone loss, that yet-unpublished data prove that estrogen therapy leads to fewer fractures in postmenopausal women and that the risk of death from endometrial cancer is less than the risk of death from disabling hip fractures. (Before accepting this latter opinion, the results of carefully controlled epidemiological studies wherein estrogen therapy is compared with other forms of treatment must be weighed.)

"There is no question that the menopausal woman and her physician face a tough decision over long-term estrogen therapy," says Dr. Lipsett. "You're dealing with probabilities and with a disease that is ten or twenty years away. Estrogen has both good and bad effects, and that's why it's so difficult to reach a conclusion about what you should do and why we say the risks and benefits have to be discussed between the patient and the physician."

To help the individual woman better understand the complexities of the disease and the reasons for advocating one or another treatment, we've asked experts from both sides to present their arguments. One speaks in favor and one against the routine and long-term use of estrogen to prevent osteoporosis.

Gilbert S. Gordan, M.D., Ph.D., began his scientific research into osteoporosis at Massachusetts General Hospital under the direction of

Dr. Albright. On his return to the University of California, San Francisco (UCSF), in 1943, he began a study on prevention of fractures in postmenopausal women with severe, far-advanced osteoporosis. Six years later Dr. Gordan established the Bone and Stone Clinic at UCSF, where he is professor of medicine. Since 1975, Dr. Gordan has been advocating low-dose, long-term estrogen replacement for the prevention of postmenopausal osteoporosis in ethnically predisposed women.

"Look at the catastrophes that occur to women as a result of losing bone. You can walk down any street in any city in the world and see little old ladies bent over with kyphosis (excessive backward curvature of the spine or humpback) and shrunken in height because of the collapse of their vertebrae. They walk as if on eggs, with a wide base, slowly and painfully crossing intersections with the help of a cane. They become crippled, and many incur serious fractures. That means a lot of hospital and nursing-home care. This problem is getting worse every year because our population of older women at risk is growing and will continue to grow in the foreseeable future. The cost in human misery and in dollars is staggering.

"Chiefly because of studies being done in Scotland; Omaha, Nebraska; Los Angeles, California, and our own in San Francisco, California, we now know that we can prevent postmenopausal osteoporosis with very low doses of estrogen and with a number of other, newer treatments. Ten years ago we had no idea this was possible, because we didn't know how to measure bone loss in its very early stages.

"The very low doses of estrogen that are effective in preventing bone loss are lower than the doses that have been incriminated— rightly or wrongly—in causing endometrial cancer. When estrogen is prescribed and taken properly, with the doses spaced out —given in cycles of twenty-one to twenty-five days each month —and when every episode of breakthrough bleeding (bleeding that occurs when the woman is taking her estrogen pills) is thoroughly investigated by a gynecologist, there is no need to fear death by cancer as a result of estrogen therapy. Anytime a doctor prescribes a drug, he or she must consider the benefits as well as the risks. Endometrial cancer is a serious condition, but fortunately it is also one of the easiest diseases to cure, provided it is detected early. Women on estrogen treatment are usually under careful medical supervision. We should keep in mind recent vital statistical data that show that at least 15,000 women die each year in this country from osteoporotic hip fractures. This death rate is very high and is a late consequence of estrogen deficiency. But the good news is that thousands of susceptible women of all races can now be protected.

"Of course no one, least of all myself, is advocating giving estrogens, or any other form of prophylaxis (prevention) routinely to *all* postmenopausal women. Today we can identify those women at risk by simple, reliable and absolutely safe and painless methods of measuring bone mass. We know that susceptible women lose about 3 percent of their skeleton a year after menopause or oophorectomy, so, allowing for a margin of error in the measuring technique, we can tell within three years whether a woman is losing a significant amount of bone. These women can then be offered prophylactic treatment with a low dose of estrogen, or other forms of therapy.

"Most women at risk who have not taken any form of prophylaxis will continue to lose bone, in my opinion. If estrogen or a progestin is started, they will regain some of that lost bone, but will never regain it all. If a woman waits until she has osteoporotic fractures, she will then need full replacement doses of estrogen to prevent further fractures. The very small doses of estrogen are only effective for *prevention* of bone loss. That is why I emphasize prevention. Small prophylactic doses of estrogen are very safe if properly supervised.

"You have to do a lot of counseling and listening when prescribing estrogen. I usually start by saying to my patients, 'I'm going to give you this hormone, and there is controversy about it. If it isn't properly supervised and taken as prescribed, some people think it can cause cancer. I don't think estrogen causes cancer, but it can cause overgrowth of the lining of the womb (endometrial hyperplasia), which is easily mistaken for early cancer.' Then I explain our regimen, telling the patient not to take the estrogen pills for the first five to seven days each month. I tell her she may have some bleeding, just like a light period, when she is off the estrogen. And I emphasize, very strongly, that if she has *any* bleeding, even minor spotting, during the estrogen cycle, she must call me *immediately,* and I will arrange for a complete gynecologic examination. This includes microscopic examination of samples of the endometrium. At the start of treatment I also explain that prevention or treatment of postmenopausal osteoporosis requires a lifelong commitment by the patient and her doctor. If we must stop the medication, for any reason, we start another form of prophylaxis right away so that the woman does not lose the protection she has acquired.

"We are going through a strange period of cancerphobia in this country right now, so much so that real diseases can be neglected, not because of the presence of cancer but because of the fear of it. Everything has its risks as well as its benefits. We can minimize risks with careful dosage and supervision. This is what we do with estrogen. For women who cannot take this hormone because of other medical problems, or who will not take it because they have been frightened by adverse publicity, we can now offer alternate treatments, for example, progestins, 'anabolics,' calcitonin or high doses of calcium. However, none of these has been studied as long as estrogen. We have been using estrogen safely for over forty years—we have a lot of experience with it. It must also be remembered that each of the other forms of treatment also has its risks and benefits.

"I consider giving estrogen, or other treatments, to prevent bone loss in susceptible women. It is similar to preventing polio or smallpox. Crippling and painful osteoporosis and fractures are preventable and should be prevented."

Christopher Longcope, M.D., is associate professor of medicine at Boston (Massachusetts) University and senior scientist at the Worcester Foundation for Experimental Biology, Shrewsbury, Massachusetts. His research on estrogen metabolism prompts a more conservative view of the relationship between the hormone and osteoporosis. Dr. Longcope speaks against the routine use of estrogen in postmenopausal women.

"In a way, it's tougher to defend *not* putting women on estrogen than it is to defend long-term estrogen therapy (ERT) for osteoporosis. The other side of the story is much more dramatic, but it may also be too simplistic. When we start estrogen therapy, we are introducing something the consequences of which are not fully known. I do not routinely recommend estrogen for several reasons.

"For one, we don't really know what causes osteoporosis. The data linking estrogen to osteoporosis are conjectural at best. For another, we haven't found anything yet that has a major effect on new bone formation. Estrogen will slightly alter the rate at which bone disappears, but it doesn't result in new bone formation. We know that estrogen acts on uterine tissues. You can show this in the laboratory by making a culture of uterine cells and adding estrogen. There's a profound effect on tissue growth. But you can't show this with bone. If estrogen does anything to bone mass, it may do it by acting through something else, and I think it would be far better to look for that something else than to prescribe estrogen.

"In general, I believe it unwise to place postmenopausal women on estrogen. Although the risk of cancer from estrogen is a real one and should be considered, it is not the only risk. Estrogens are usually administered orally and are absorbed and go immediately through the liver at a relatively high concentration. This is a different process from the physiologic one, in which estrogen is secreted by the ovaries and doesn't circulate through the liver first. At high concentrations in the liver, estrogen can have a number of adverse effects. Estrogen increases the synthesis of clotting factors, of some lipoproteins and of transport proteins. It is through these mechanisms that the risk of heart attacks, blood clots and strokes is increased in people on estrogens. These effects were initially ascribed to oral contraceptives, but I think the type of estrogen is not as critical as the fact that the estrogen is taken orally.

"Women are sometimes urged to begin estrogen therapy at the climacteric because if they wait, the therapy may not be effective. This reasoning is largely based on a study that compared bone loss in two groups of surgically menopausal women. (One group was administered estrogen, and the other was not.) I'm not sure that it is accurate or fair to apply these data to women who experience a natural menopause. If you remove the ovaries, you remove all the steroids they produce, and the body is operating with far fewer androgens and estrogens than if the ovaries had not been removed. Also, if estrogens are effective in treating osteoporosis, the point at which treatment begins should not be quite as critical.

"The woman who is menopausal shouldn't feel she has to rush

off and start taking estrogen. Women who have a large bone mass to begin with probably needn't be concerned nearly as much as small, frail women whose bone mass is low. These latter are the ones who should be watched carefully. Women with a family history of osteoporosis should also be followed closely. I would advise women such as these to be sure to maintain an adequate calcium intake, to be sure their vitamin D intake is adequate, to restrict their alcohol intake, to stop smoking and to maintain a reasonable degree of activity. These are measures that can be taken with safety and yet can be of great benefit to the patient. I would save estrogen and other types of treatment, such as fluoride, until the positive effects of such therapies are more clear-cut.

"I certainly don't see any reason for women to panic. There's a lot of research being done in the area of osteoporosis, using techniques that were not known a few years ago. And we are continually getting new information. From recent research we are learning more about the causes of osteoporosis. When we know the causes, we'll know more about treating the problem. It may be that within a few years something will come along to totally change our views on estrogen therapy, and we will discover that a completely innocuous substance can be given to all women that will keep their bone mass adequate. I am optimistic about the future. For the present, I think women in their late forties and fifties should follow the simple regimens that I've described, which carry less risk than estrogen therapy."

The Male Climacteric

When Gretzinger and Dege began their search for families willing to talk about menopause, they found a few men who seemed unusually eager to participate in the study. "Later we learned why," says Gretzinger. "They thought we were going to talk about male menopause."

Male menopause. It has been called myth, termed a synonym for mid-life crisis and rejected out of hand, even in some modern medical texts. But in general the phenomenon is receiving ever-growing recognition. Only the words are misleading.

Women experience dramatic and regular shifts in hormonal

balance throughout their active reproductive years. Men, too, are believed to experience some cyclic fluctuation in hormone production, though the changes are considered to be minimal. For the man there is no menopause, no cessation of menses. Instead the male body undergoes a slight but steady decrease in hormonal output. For most men, the change is negligible and generally accompanied by a gentle tapering off of sexual desire and performance—not enough to bother most. But some men do experience a dramatic shift in hormone balance. This condition affects only a small percentage of the male population between the ages of forty-one and sixty and is known as the male climacteric. Unlike menopause, which is a natural process, the climacteric is considered an illness.

Herbert S. Kupperman, M.D., has spent two decades studying the male climacteric. Dr. Kupperman, associate professor of medicine at New York University Medical Center, explains the phenomenon:

First, the male climacteric is defined as the physiological cessation of testicular function.

Second, it has three symptoms: a loss of potency, which can be either premature ejaculation or inability to have an erection; hot flashes, similar to but generally less severe than those associated with menopausal women; and a tendency to be nervous, indecisive in actions and prone to angry outbursts. In some instances, the signs appear suddenly, but in most cases the climacteric is such an insidious, slowly developing condition that a man may easily shrug off his concern or attribute the symptoms to other factors. Being "on edge" can easily be associated with mid-life changes and conflicts. Hot flashes can be rationalized away or attributed to colds, flu or a virus that seems to be going around. Sexual impotency may be linked to stress or overwork. Although psychological rather than organic problems account for most of these complaints in males over forty years old, physiological causes should not be ruled out.

In a recent study, researchers from Harvard Medical School, Boston, Massachusetts, screened 105 impotent men, who ranged in age from eighteen to seventy-five and had endured potency problems for six months to thirty years. In thirty-seven of these cases, endocrine imbalance was found to be the cause of the men's difficulties. In these patients, the problems were traced to abnormalities in either the hypothalamus, pituitary gland, testes or thyroid. In thirty-three of the men, androgenic hormone replacement therapy with the hormone testosterone quickly restored potency. Furthermore, once treated, the men felt better in general. Their sense of well-being was improved, as well as their ability to have erections, engage in sex and experience normal libido.

One case in point is Richard Verons, a middle-aged man who had been impotent for eleven years before becoming a subject of the study. Richard was born with a cryptorchid left testicle, a relatively common condition in which one testicle remains lodged in the abdominal cavity and does not descend into the scrotum. Twelve years later, this man's testicle was brought down by surgical means, but it was already atrophied and unable to produce testosterone. Nevertheless, Richard was able to function sexually. He married, fathered a child and had no potency problems until around age forty, when his functioning testicle began to fail.

Richard noticed that the testicle was becoming smaller. Then he began having problems getting erections. He sought medical care and for eleven years was unsuccessfully treated for psychogenically based impotence. During this time, his marriage broke up, and the patient became increasingly depressed and disappointed in himself.

At age fifty-one, Richard joined the Boston study. His problem was diagnosed as gonadal failure that resulted in a very low level of testosterone production. Hormone replacement therapy restored the man to full potency. His self-image has improved, he has begun dating steadily and even talks of possible marriage.

At this point, there are two schools of thought concerning the impact of hormone imbalance on male potency. Some physicians feel that the problem must be consistent and sustained. They argue that if a man complains of sexual dysfunction with his wife but can perform with another woman or gets an erection while watching an erotic movie, he is not in the climacteric, says Dr. Kupperman. Others, however, maintain that hormone deficiency can exist even when a man is occasionally potent. "We have seen individuals who've had sporadic erections, some who even claimed to have been occasionally successful sexually who we know are hypogonadotropic, that is, their gonads are not producing testosterone," explains Richard F. Spark, M.D., who headed the Harvard study.

Middle-aged men who are experiencing impotence should seek counsel with their physician, who may suggest that medical tests be taken. One of the tests he or she may prescribe measures testosterone levels, which, in climacteric males, are markedly decreased. Another measures gonadotropic levels, which may be dramatically elevated. In addition, levels of the hormone prolactin are measured. (Prolactin is produced by the pituitary gland.) Too much prolactin indicates a possible microadenoma, a small benign tumor, affecting the pituitary. In these patients, medication and/or surgery may restore normal potency.

When androgenic hormone therapy is instituted, such treatment becomes lifelong and may involve side effects, such as breast tenderness and water retention, which can increase blood pressure. Ironically, just as estrogen therapy is associated with endometrial cancer in women, so too—at least in theory—is androgenic hormone therapy potentially linked to prostate cancer in men. Dr. Kupperman, however, who has treated more than 300 men for the climacteric, reports not a single incidence of prostatic cancer among his patients. For some men hormone therapy is not recommended. These include men with histories of prostatic cancer, high blood pressure, congestive heart failure or marked edema or swelling. Men undergoing the therapy are urged to have regular physical checkups and routine prostate exams, as well as prostatic acid phosphatase tests to help diagnose prostatic cancer early.

Hormone therapy can lead to dramatic improvements for the man in the male climacteric, says Dr. Kupperman. "The worst thing a man can do if he's having any of these problems is to think that they are all in his head and to ignore them."

8

THE MIDDLE-AGED PERSON AND THE FAMILY

"Sometimes I feel I'm standing on a beach of shifting sand. There are moments when everything in my life is stable, then suddenly I feel something start to give way, and I wonder, 'What now. Will I be able to handle it?' " The woman who made this comment is fifty-two years old. "Nothing is really overwhelming," she explains. "It's just that there is so much change, everywhere." Her list runs a wide course: changes in personal expectations and dreams, changes in her husband's perception of work and career, changes in herself as a now-menopausal woman.

And there is more to come.

For rising in the not-too-distant future is the certainty of changes in her family, too. "You get used to a certain status quo. I guess you fall into the trap of thinking life is always going to be like that, so it's unsettling, sometimes even scary, to think there's more of the unpredictable coming and that it's going to hit so close to home."

On a beach of shifting sand, all the possibilities have to be considered: the impact of children leaving home, the altered relationship with one's aging parents, the chance for renewal in the long-time marriage, the increasing threat of divorce; the likelihood that death might claim a spouse and play its own cruel game with an individual's future. (Widowhood and widowerhood are discussed in Chapter 9.)

"I'm basically optimistic," said the woman we spoke with. "I have faith in myself and belief in tomorrow. I think it can be good, but I don't think it's necessarily going to be easy. I can only learn from myself and from other people who are going through the same thing. Cheers to us all!"

Marriage at Mid-Life

Louise and Tom Keane have been married for twenty-five years. They have spent a quarter of a century together, and during this time they have witnessed the seemingly never-ending cycles of change and stability that characterize so much of human existence. They have moved easily, though not without their own personal pain, from one plateau to another. Now they stand ready for a step that will take them almost full circle to the point where it all began, in the Mississippi River town where they first met and married. Like other long-married, middle-aged couples, Tom and Louise Keane must prepare themselves for a new life. In a few years, the last of the Keanes' four children will have left home. The front door will open and close less frequently, the stereo will play quieter tunes, the garage will be less cluttered. Louise and Tom wonder what they'll talk about with the kids gone. They agree that work will fill in much of the space, but even that has a temporariness about it now that never existed before. Tom, a psychiatric social worker at a local hospital, faces early retirement in four years, when he's fifty-nine, or routine retirement in seven years, at age sixty-two.

Louise is a registered nurse at the same hospital. She had worked before marriage, dropped out for eleven years to rear the children and has been back at work full-time for fourteen years. She toys with the idea of working part-time at some point, perhaps soon.

Meanwhile, the future is full of questions. "I don't think we're prepared in any way for when the kids leave," says Louise, though she already has a mental list of activities lined up. Tom is more tentative. He has thought of spending time at the new parish hall, but is unsure about what he'll do. He entertains the idea of becoming a free-of-charge psychotherapist for the community, but wonders if he'll ever honestly want to see another patient or hear about another problem.

"We need to find things we can do together or with other

people," says Louise. "When the kids were young and were in scouting, our friends were the other scout leaders. Then for many years we went to family camp and had a good relationship with the people there. Maybe we could renew those friendships, but we're just not doing it right now."

At this point the Keanes are not even sure if they will stay in their present location. Both have dismissed the thought of returning to their hometown because "it wouldn't be the same," but have thought little beyond that. "We have enough money, basically, to do whatever we would want," says Tom, though the possibility exists that their children or Louise's parents, both of whom are still living, will need financial help in the future.

All this is peripheral, however, to the fundamental, underlying question: What is going to happen to Tom and Louise's relationship and to the marriage, the foundation that lies buried under twenty-five years of daily existence and acquired routine?

"I wonder about this sometimes," says Tom, "but I just don't know. I'm aware that I should be thinking and planning, but I haven't really done it yet." He admits that he's been preoccupied with the children and their academic achievements, which to him are crucial. "In a sense, they are more important than our relationship," he explains, and Louise agrees, with some qualification. "For you more so than for me," she says. "You are more concerned about the kids than I am. I think it's time they got on with their own lives."

Tom also acknowledges that when he does focus on the future, he tends to do so with calculator in hand and with his mind tuned to the economics of retirement. "There is more risk in growing old today than there was a generation ago," he argues. "So you have to have more data and plans." In the next breath, he challenges his own line of reasoning and wonders if it's not just a way of avoiding having to think about the other issues.

"When I do project ahead, I say, 'It'll be fine.' Just like twenty-five years ago. You and me together. It will be better than before. But then, I really don't know what it will be like. There are no guarantees, are there?" Tom looks quietly at his wife. "You know, we really had very little time together alone in the beginning. We were married for a year, and then the children came. We really had little time to get to know each other. Now, do we approach each other in an adventuresome and exciting way, or do we level off into a week-in and week-out blasé kind of existence? I guess it could go either way."

"After twenty-five years of marriage you do get into a bit of a rut," says Louise. "The daily conversation tends to be the same: Weather, kids, how your day went, that sort of thing. We haven't had much real fun lately. We don't go out together very often, and there's something special about doing that. I think we've grown apart some, but not seriously. Basically our relationship is good enough, and I think we can build on it. But we have to be aware that we have to do that or else we could continue to go our separate ways. But I think it can be fun, if we work at it."

For a moment neither one speaks. They are caught up in thoughts of past and present and thoughts of the future. Finally, Tom begins again, and the words come slowly, spoken from the heart. When he finishes, both he and his wife smile, as if recognizing the intrinsic value and truth in what he has said. "People at this age do need to ask themselves, 'What did I like about this person and what do I like still? What are the positives that are still there and can be used to build upon and make something even better?' It isn't too difficult for people to find the negatives and to ignore the positives. I think the responsibilities of life tend to dampen the sparkle you have inside. But they haven't killed it. Maybe I could have fun and enjoy life again. Maybe all these years later, after the burdens of work, children and home are finished, maybe I could still become a more interesting person to you."

The Empty Nest

Of all the changes in family relationships facing mid-life couples like Louise and Tom Keane, perhaps the least traumatic is the one involving children and their departure from home—the literal emptying of the nest. Recent theories have painted this as a dismal period for the wife and mother, a neutral one for the husband and father and a largely negative time for the marriage relationship itself. In fact, Louise and Tom Keane's attitudes toward the empty nest are more representative of the typical parental reaction. Like Louise, women often breathe a sigh of relief. Like Tom, men who are thought to be immune to this departure are genuinely affected and touched by a sense of loss. Overall, however, the empty nest is not the end of the world for the majority of modern men and women.

Empty nest merely means the kids are gone. It encompasses a nebulous time frame that revolves around this final departure from home. The empty nest can begin and end with the last good-bye as the youngest walks out the door, suitcases in hand, or it can endure for as long as it takes for the kids to establish themselves successfully in marriage or a career. Of itself, the empty nest is neither positive nor negative. But add the word *syndrome,* and the situation changes. Suddenly parents are thought to have predictable and often enduring problems coping with the loss or leaving of their children.

The primary characteristic of the empty-nest syndrome (ENS) is a sense of loss of identity (Who am I now?). Added to that are a lack of behavioral norms and role models (What am I supposed to do now? What are the guidelines for my behavior?) as well as depression or a sense of loss and sadness. "Actually, we don't have any support for the syndrome as a large-scale phenomenon," says Dolores Cabic Borland, Ph.D., assistant professor in the department of family and child ecology at Michigan State University, East Lansing. "I'm concerned that by talking about it and splashing it across headlines we may create the expectation, and then people will begin looking for it to happen to them."

The most recent data available support this idea. In a San Francisco survey, for example, 160 women were questioned about their reactions to the empty nest. Only one experienced the classical symptoms of the syndrome. For the others, the departure was welcomed with a mix of emotions and even, more importantly, was recognized as a transitional and temporary period.

Half the parents interviewed in a Colorado State University, Fort Collins, study felt that launching the children fulfilled one of their parental goals. Even more said the event was beneficial: It brought relief from worry and responsibility for the children, a new sense of freedom, an improved marital state and better relationships with the kids. For these parents, the empty nest was most difficult if children were considered too young to leave home or if the departure coincided with another major mid-life change, such as retirement, job shift or menopause. Researchers from the

University of California, Los Angeles, and Duke University, Durham, North Carolina, have found that the empty nest is least traumatic for people in their fifties because they are ready for children to leave and perceive this as a "normal" event for that time in their lives.

It is important to realize that the very concept of the empty nest is relatively new in our society. At the turn of the century, for example, families were normally not "emptied" when children left home. Instead, boarders were brought in to fill up space and help out economically. When the Depression hit, many children came back to live at home again, and those who left did not move far away.

Today, one could hypothesize that if the empty nest is a problem for anyone, says Dr. Borland, it may be for the generation of women now in mid-life. The generation of women before them had less time to think about the departure of children from the home. They were too busy either filling wartime industrial jobs or baby-sitting grandchildren so that younger mothers could become Rosie the Riveters. The current generation of women in their fifties are the ones who, as young women, came home to suburbia when the men came home from the war.

These women did what society dictated: They focused all their energies and attention on husband and children. They are the women who did not pursue careers outside their families, who were told they had only one place and that was in the home. Now, with their children gone, they need to find new responsibilities and a new purpose. Those who succeed in creating a new life for themselves experience little trauma. But for many of these women, the transition may be difficult. For them the empty nest may represent a painful loss.

The women best equipped to handle the empty nest are women, like Louise Keane, who have developed additional interests and responsibilities outside the home. If you have extra activities, if you work outside the home, you are at an advantage. But if you do not, you can take positive steps now that will help you to deal successfully with the empty nest.

First, face up to the fact that your children will mature and leave home. Keep track of the time and energy you devote to activities, such as meal preparation and housekeeping, that revolve around your children. Then imagine how time allocated for these tasks will wind down when your children are gone. Anticipating these kinds of very real changes in your life-style will help you begin preparing for them.

Second, ask yourself what else you can do or will want to do with your newfound free time. It is important for you honestly to assess your feelings and needs and to explore your options. If you are interested in volunteer work, for example, you should determine what avenues are open to you. Check with local women's groups about their activities; learn if area hospitals or schools use volunteers. The more information you have about available positions, the easier it will be for you to decide what it is you want to do.

If you are interested in working at a paid job, start now to study the employment market and to evaluate your skills. There are women's centers in nearly every city that can provide helpful information; check your library for appropriate guides and directories. No matter who you are, no matter what your educational background or economic status, no matter where you live, you have viable options that you can pursue. (In Chapter 15, we show how some middle-aged men and women have reshaped their lives; what they have learned can provide valuable information and insight for you.) Remember, the sooner you begin to investigate the possibilities that are open to you, the easier it will be for you to cope with the transition you will experience when your children leave home.

Caring for Aging Parents

Louise Keane's children range in age from eighteen to twenty-three; they are young, healthy, well educated and generally prepared to take on the world. Their mother is optimistic about their opportunities and future.

Louise's parents are eighty-three. They, too, are healthy and self-sufficient. Louise speaks of them confidently and yet with some qualification. "If something should happen . . ." she says, and then she hesitates a moment. "One sister lives nearby and is very close to them. She helps out. There are five of us, and we would share any responsibility. I don't think we would have to alter any of our plans." Left unspoken are the possibilities that this situation might change in some unforeseeable way and, in fact, alter many of Louise's and Tom's plans.

Take the example of Kay and Fred Torshaw. Kay had worked for an airline company, Fred for a railway firm. Once the children were gone, the Torshaws planned to utilize job-related travel privileges and see the world, first in small doses and later, after retirement, on longer jaunts. Then Kay's mother, a widow, had a severe stroke, and her care became a top priority. Now Kay and Fred, still dreaming of travel, stay close to home and handle the primary responsibility of caring for the elderly woman.

In another instance, a middle-aged woman and her husband spend $1,000 each month to ensure the wife's widowed mother a tiny apartment in a retirement hotel. The stories are endless. A professor at a large university built a small home for his parents, then arranged with his wife to take separate vacations because someone always had to be around to "look after" the aging couple. One middle-aged couple quit their jobs, sold the family home and bought an old two-story structure. They opened an art gallery downstairs and built loft living quarters upstairs for themselves, with a separate attached apartment for the wife's parents. Another man went to court to fight the zoning rule in his suburb that prohibited him from providing a similar living arrangement in his own home for his elderly mother.

"The big problem right now is that middle-aged people didn't expect this [caring for aging parents] to happen to them," explains Ethel Shanas, Ph.D., professor of sociology at the University of Illinois, Chicago Circle Campus. "They thought they would raise their children and then be free. Women say, 'I never thought when I got to this age that I would have to worry about my parents. Now is the time for my husband and me to be free to do things together, but we're not.' "

Adult children must usually cope with three basic problem areas in dealing with their elderly parents. First, they may have to provide financial support and health care. (The adult child may be directly responsible for providing this aid or simply serve as the person who arranges for the needed help.) Second, middle-aged children often must learn to become information givers. They are their parents' link to a bureaucratic world that may be unfamiliar to the elderly. Aged parents often need someone to negotiate the system for them. They need someone who knows who to call, what to say, how to get the foot in the door. It might take a dozen phone calls to get the information on a needed service. The elderly may not be willing to persist through all those calls. Someone may have to assist them, and that someone is likely to be the middle-aged child.

Finally adult children must grapple with the psychological problems imposed by the changing parent-child relationship: the denial of anticipated freedom, the strain of having to be an adult yourself while still remaining a child in the parent's eyes, the pressure of having to compete with your own parents for the attention of your own children, the temptation to give more help than is needed and wanted, resentment at being responsible for elderly in-laws whom you never lived near and hardly know or who may have objected to your marriage to their child, anger at feeling that too much is expected of you and guilt because you feel you are not doing enough or because you've been forced to place a parent in a nursing home.

Since couples, even the very elderly, tend to look after each other, the situation is often more critical for adult children if only one parent is surviving. Usually, it is the mother. In that case, says Dr. Shanas, it makes a big difference if she has either worked all her life or, at least, since her middle age. "By age sixty-five, the woman who has worked outside the home tends to be in better health, is more active and has more interests than the woman who has not. This has implications for the middle-aged couple, because trying to plan with the older mother who has worked and done things on her own is different from trying to plan with the mother whose focus of activity has been the home. It is almost as if the older population of women is composed of two different groups of people."

If your parents are still living, you should begin now to plan for the possibility that one day you may have to care for them. Although each family's situation is unique, there are similar problems to consider. These include the following:

• *Housing.* You must face the fact that one day your parents may not be able to live independently. There are questions you should ask of yourself: Should they move in with you? Or should you make other, more appropriate arrangements? Retirement hotels and communities are becoming increasingly popular. It is a good idea to become familiar with the resources in your area. Perhaps your parents live in a distant city. Will they be willing to move to your community, or can arrangements be made for them to remain in a familiar setting? What are the possibilities? What are the costs?

• *Medical care.* In addition to the care provided by your parents' personal physician, an increasing number of services are available that provide needed medical care to the elderly on an at-home basis. Check with your doctor and local community health center to find out what services are available in your area. Talk with representatives from your hospital's social service department and from a local nursing-care agency to learn about costs and availability of at-home assistance.

It is possible that you may have to consider a nursing home for an elderly parent. Not all nursing homes are alike. Services vary, as do costs. Ask your physician for guidance in determining how much care your parent needs. Talk to neighbors and friends about their experiences with different facilities and be sure to visit the nursing homes in your area.

• *Activities.* You will do both yourself and your parents a service if you become familiar with the senior-citizens groups in your community. Many provide a variety of programs for the elderly. Having something to do and having friends to talk with will help your parents maintain a sense of independence and will lessen the demands they make on your time and energy. For information, check with local social service organizations, watch newspaper announcements, call your local office of senior citizens and talk with your neighbors about the resources with which they are familiar.

There are no hard-and-fast rules for you to follow in determining how you can best aid your parents. But you can facilitate decision making and help ease tensions by following these guidelines:

First, start now to talk to your parents about the future. If they bring up the topics of possible widowhood, altered living arrangements and decreasing independence, listen to them. If they don't initiate the conversation, then you should.

Second, include your parents in all decisions. Never make decisions for them; even if you make the proper choice, they might resent being left out.

Third, share responsibilities with other family members. If you do not provide direct care, offer indirect support to the siblings who are caring for your parents. Make regular phone calls or write letters to your parents; contribute to their financial support; arrange for the direct-care givers to take regular vacations or to have regular days or nights out. If you are the person responsible for direct care, let other family members know that they must assist you.

Fourth, learn to utilize the resources at hand and don't be afraid to try something that has not been done before. If your mother wants to live alone, for example, but cannot deal with marketing or other errands, hire a teenager to help her. Tailor your solutions to your family's particular wants and needs. Remember, too, that family histories vary tremendously. What works for a close-knit, amicable family won't apply in a situation where no one has been on friendly terms for years.

Finally, says Dr. Shanas, you should avoid thinking of the aging parent strictly as a problem that requires a solution. Many of the elderly have much to offer in terms of insight, experience and wisdom. They can be loving and your own close companions— if you let them.

Changing Attitudes toward Marriage and Divorce

In the 1950s, when Louise and Tom Keane exchanged their wedding vows, a basic philosophical change was occurring in the Western world, one that would eventually reach deep into the roots of marriage itself. Existentialism, a belief in the overriding value of the immediate moment, and the humanistic movement, a faith in the power of the individual over his or her own fate, blended together to alter the way people looked at themselves and at the institutions surrounding them. Marriage was no exception. Prior to World War II, marriage was highly structured and hierarchical. Society, church and civil law made the rules and imposed them on the populace. These rules dictated the form and nature of marriage, paying only lip service to content. The revolutionary change in philosophy loosened the hold and also shifted the focus away from appearance and conformity and onto content. People began to demand as a right a small slice of heaven on earth, a chance at personal happiness and fulfillment. They also began to assume more direct responsibility for their own well-being. In terms of marriage, they asked for openness and quality, intimacy and an avenue for growth. "He's a good provider" and "My dinner is on the table at six" began to fade as the criteria for an acceptable spouse. People wanted more, and, through this, marriage evolved into what is called a companionship relationship.

People like Louise and Tom began to view the married state as a means toward personal gratification. Those in mid-life today were in the vanguard of the marriage revolution. They were the first wave of a new direction, inundated at one end by the old values that dictated that marriage remain solvent for the sake of the children and for the sake of society, and intrigued at the other by the tantalizing prospect of personal happiness. Suddenly, they are told by society and by their peers that if marriage does not measure up, they can get out. The problem is that few people have told them how marriage can be made to work under the new rules and expectations.

The middle-aged couple today that wants a companionship relationship has no models. The next generation, looking back to them for a model, sees more disaster than success. One in five marriages ends in divorce in the middle years. Only 10 percent of those that remain undisrupted are considered really good, strong unions. Virtually every survey of modern marriages supports the idea of disenchantment and decline in marital satisfaction in the middle years. Something happens along the way to lessen the attraction, diminish the rewards and increase the distance between the two who began a life together with only the highest of expectations.

In a study of 138 people divorced in their middle years, conducted by the University of Oklahoma, Norman, the majority said that their marriages had started out positively, had remained that way during the early years and then had gradually declined. The intangible factor that determined the success or failure of the union was the *quality* of the relationship as perceived by both husband and wife. Tom Keane expressed basically this idea when he said to his wife, "I can no longer think of you as the mother of four children and myself as the father of four kids. Now you're Louise, my wife, a female person and I am Tom, husband, and a male person, and what does all that mean? Certainly not the same thing as ten years ago, when you were mommy and I was daddy. We have to explore the positives again, the things that used to make for happy times." If they don't, reasoned Tom, they will simply level off in their relationship. "I don't want to live like that, though I probably could. It wouldn't be fair to you or to me, but we could just settle for it." What Tom is seeking is companionship and intimacy. According to a study done at the University of California at San Francisco, his dream is no different from that of other middle-aged couples.

Marriage counselors are and have been available to couples needing help and guidance. But to consult a counselor implied that the marriage was in trouble, and to admit this was always humiliating and disgraceful. If people did eventually go for counseling, they were often too late and too alienated from each other to gather the motivation for reconstructing their relationship. Today, another approach exists, one that quietly developed in tandem with the marriage revolution. The concept is called marriage enrichment and currently is offered by some twenty different national organizations. (For information about programs in your area, contact the local library or ask at your place of worship.)

After many years of marriage, it is very easy to take your spouse for granted. Marriage enrichment tries to counter this tendency. The primary goal of the movement is to stimulate an underlying level of intimate rapport or communication, to create the type of relationship the couple may have had while they were courting or in the early days of their marriage. "We try to get people to see the importance of communication on a meaningful level on a regular, daily basis," explains Father Thoralf Thielen, the clergy person on the executive team of National Marriage Encounter, St. Paul, Minnesota. "We don't mean talking just about problems or about routine things such as buying a new car or recarpeting the house; rather the point is getting the other to know your hopes and fears about almost everything in life: its physical, mental, emotional, spiritual, social and religious aspects. You need to tell each other not just what you *think* but how you *feel*. Are you angry, happy, sad, upset or shy—to let the other person know what is going on inside you."

Typically, marriage enrichment programs offer married couples an escape from a routine setting and provide the chance for them to see each other in a new light. Home, children and work problems are left behind. Sessions are designed to show couples how much they might not even know about each other. In one session, for example, participants are asked the types of questions that will help them reveal something about their inner selves. At one meeting, a woman was asked, "How do you feel about walking in the rain?" Her sentimental response surprised her husband. Here was a more gentle, introspective woman than he had realized. The session taught him something about his wife that he had not known.

Communication on this level takes the boredom out of a relationship, says Father Thielen. It helps you develop a real sense of life and love and growth. "Communication based on friendship and trust and a desire to love leads to unity, and if you have unity, you are going to have happiness, even if there are problems to deal with. It's when you have separation and division that you have pain."

It is true, however, that talking about communication is much easier than actually doing it. Couples who attend marriage enrichment programs claim they have no time at home for private, intimate conversations. Another deterrent to intimacy and communication is lack of self-esteem. "If you think of yourself as a zero, how can you ask anyone to love you? You have to find out who you are and what you have to offer first," says Father Thielen. In the Marriage Encounter program, the first step is self-encounter. The idea is to learn to get in touch with yourself first, literally to discover yourself, your feelings and ideas and your own value and dignity as a person, before reaching out to the other person. "I never worked so hard to find out what my feelings were," said one middle-aged man after a Marriage Encounter weekend, "but it's nice to know they were there."

In the marriage enrichment setting, couples also learn to deal constructively with conflict. "Our honeyed concepts of romantic love imply that you must not be angry with someone you love. If you are, it's considered terrible. In fact, it's entirely normal," says David Mace, Ph.D., co-founder of the Association for Couples in Marriage Enrichment (ACME), Winston-Salem, North Carolina. "We now know that conflict is an integral part of marriage. If skillfully used, it can lead to further growth in a relationship. If you ignore it or just fight about it, you achieve nothing."

Unfortunately, many couples have a problem with old, unresolved conflicts that have never been put to rest and that keep popping up, often years after the triggering incident. For these individuals, a marriage enrichment weekend may not be sufficient. They may need special counseling. "These are people in what we call yo-yo marriages," says Dr. Mace. "Whenever they try to get close, they only reactivate the conflicts they have never settled. They move apart again, then come back together and so on. People do this for a time. Eventually they find themselves living together but emotionally distant from each other, or they separate and may even divorce."

Divorce at Mid-Life

Increasingly, many middle-aged couples are choosing divorce. In 1964, more than a million and a half divorces were granted to people over the age of forty-five. In ten years, the figure doubled. If expert predictions are correct, the rate is tripling right now. That means that by the late 1980s, one half of all the married men and women over forty-five will agree to end their marriages. Although divorce is easier to obtain and imposes less social stigma than ever before, the breakup of a long-time marriage can still be one of the most difficult experiences an individual has ever had to deal with. For the middle-aged man or woman, the situation becomes even more critical.

"Those of us who are middle-aged have a life script calling for us to marry and live happily ever after," says Sharon Helm, Ph.D., psychologist, relationship counselor and director of the Assertive Training Institute, Kansas City, Missouri. "The decision to divorce is in total conflict with this idea. Psychologically we are just *not* prepared for it."

A Case Study in Divorce: One Woman's Story

Anne Carson, fifty-three, was divorced six months ago, after twenty-eight years of marriage. On the surface, she says, her marriage looked perfect. Her husband, Jay, was a corporate vice-president and an active community leader. She was the model wife and mother of four children who kept busy after the kids were grown with a part-time job selling children's clothes, for "pin money." The Carsons owned the obligatory two cars and the comfortable suburban home. They belonged to the country club and for years were seen at all the right functions, all the proper places.

On the inside, things were different. Jay expressed little interest in the children and shared no common activities with his wife. There were no family picnics, no real vacations, except to Jay's hometown to visit his mother. From the beginning, he left the running of the home and family to his wife and made his own rules for himself, always allotting for evenings out with the boys and for summer weekends on the golf course. When their youngest child, still an infant, was hospitalized in a special medical center for children, Jay made the ninety-mile round trip twice in six months. Anne went every day. When she got home, nerves jangled and with three youngsters waiting for her attention, she'd fix a drink to calm herself. Within six years, she had quarts of vodka hidden around the house and, though sober all day long, drank herself into oblivion almost every evening. The only exceptions were the times she accompanied Jay to work-related affairs and, for his sake, "behaved."

Six years ago Anne joined Alcoholics Anonymous (AA) and hasn't had a drink since. Five years ago, her husband took up with another woman, a divorced mother with six children, the same age as Anne. Three years ago he completely stopped having sexual relations with his wife. Yet when Jay asked for a divorce, Anne was overwhelmed.

"We didn't fight. I was always the type to keep everything inside me. We didn't even fight over her. I knew about her, but I could have gone on forever. I loved the man and blamed myself for the problems. I was raised to think the husband was king. And I wasn't really unhappy. I had just accepted this as my lot in life. I thought we'd get along, that he would be content with having his laundry done and his breakfast on the table."

It was Jay's suggestion that Anne file for a divorce. "It would look better that way," he told her. Don't worry about alimony either, he said, because he would always look after her. "Let's make it a friendly divorce." And Anne did.

She made no charge of adultery, didn't push to disprove his claim that he had no money, though she had good reason to believe otherwise, and didn't fight for maintenance payments. "I didn't want to make him mad because I kept hoping he would come back," she explains, but now she is bitter. "You'd think twenty-eight years would count for something. Not just a pat on the back."

Anne is plagued by financial worry. She came away from the divorce with a new condominium for herself and her youngest daughter, but with little else. She works full-time now, but her weekly take-home pay is not much. "I have to get a better job, but I need more training first, that's why I signed up for a typing course. I need more money. I need something to stimulate my mind. I am desperately afraid of what will happen to me if I should get sick. Would he help? I don't know." Recently, Anne asked Jay if he could pay a $28 monthly health insurance fee not included under her job. He said no.

In the first few months after the divorce, Anne would use any excuse to catch a glimpse of her former husband. Even now she still dreams of him nightly, still thinks of him constantly. "I don't know how to divorce myself from him, how to turn my mind off." And she would take him back in an instant, even while recognizing that she is fighting a losing battle. Before, no matter where Jay was, she knew that eventually he would come home. Now she must get used to the idea that he will never be back again.

Anne refuses to live her life through her children. Since most of her friends are still married, socializing with them is often difficult. "I would love to go out just for dinner or a movie," she says. "I miss that terribly. But how to go about meeting eligible men, I just don't know." AA remains necessary for Anne, although now she is considering divorce counseling as well. "I guess the problem is that I still think of myself as married."

What should you do if you are involved in the divorce process? Put practicality foremost, says Dr. Helm, then think about emotional needs. She suggests the following:

• First, arrange financial matters. Decide where you will live and how much money you will need. Think about where the money will come from.

• Second, decide what you will do with your life. Can you keep working? Do you need to find a job? Who can assist you?

It's important for you to establish contact with an outside individual or group you can go to for advice and counsel. Friends don't always work in this respect, because they are too involved with their own interests. The resource people you seek out should have nothing to gain or lose from the decisions you make. Middle-aged women have to assume, perhaps for the first time, the responsibility for taking the initiative in their lives, something they may not even know how to do.

• Third, analyze how the divorce will influence your place in the family structure and how it will affect your social network and your friendships. You must be realistic and face the fact that divorce often disrupts old relationships.

Some of the most difficult problems you will face after a divorce revolve around socializing and sexual behavior. After years of marriage, you may not know how to face a social situation alone. You may need help in learning how to initiate a relationship. Literally, this can come down to "What do you say after you've said hello?" You may also be confused about or overwhelmed by the matter of sex. Morals have changed since you were single. It is not unreasonable that you aren't sure of the rules and may be bothered with embarrassment and even guilt.

If you do not learn how to deal with these problems, you can become increasingly isolated. There is a danger that you will build a cocoon of emptiness and just sit there, secure but alone, safe but unhappy. If this happens, then it may become more difficult for you to establish new relationships.

It is critical that you not avoid these issues after a divorce, says Dr. Helm. If you are experiencing problems, you should seek help, either from counselors, friends or a peer group.

You also must take the time to nurture yourself. Nurturing means being nice to yourself in a way that's important to you, whether this involves taking a vacation or indulging in a new activity.

Most importantly, you must try to avoid getting caught up in the anger or "poor-me" stage of divorce. Such feelings are normal for a short-term period, especially if genuine financial or socialization problems are involved, but they become destructive if they drag on for months.

"At some point, it is necessary to get over yourself, to get to the point where you stop hurting yourself," says Dr. Helm. Unfortunately we tend to think that if we do that, we are not dealing with the genuine pain we should be feeling. Many of us seem to function as if we have an incredible quota of pain we are supposed to feel. To a large degree it is optional. When is enough, enough? Ultimately we each make that decision for ourselves, and we can make it two weeks earlier if we choose.

A Case Study in Divorce: One Man's Story

Frank Riley, divorced now for five years, is past the "hurting" stages caused by the breakup of his marriage and past feeling responsible for everything that went wrong. But he still remembers the shock of hearing his wife of twenty years, Helen, tell him that she was getting nothing from their marriage and that if things didn't improve, she wanted out. "She said she felt enslaved and had no freedom, that her role of mother was one of drudgery. I was overwhelmed by that. She could have worked if she wanted to. I never said she had to stay home with the kids."

All through their marriage Frank thought he and his wife had communicated well, had understood where the other was and how the other felt. Suddenly he found out differently. He had communicated; his wife had not.

In the long, often torturous year they spent trying to keep their relationship together, Frank learned for the first time of things he had done that had hurt his wife. He learned, too, of other instances when decisions were made that she felt had been his entirely. And he found out that all their long talks had been his long talks, about topics that were important only to him. "For years, I wondered what I had done to cause this woman such pain," he said. "Finally I concluded she had done it to herself. She knew when she did something to anger me, because I told her. I told her what bothered me, but she never gave me back the same information. We used to go around and around on decisions. Then she would leave them to me, and I think now that I operated pretty straight on the basis of the information I had."

The months before the decision to divorce were filled with tension and conflict. Helen had an affair, openly, and urged her husband to do the same. He protested, but she insisted and even found a partner for him. It lasted three weeks, says Frank, and was the most unsatisfactory relationship he had ever had. Meanwhile, he and Helen were talking, twenty-four hours a day, it seemed. He was accused of sloughing off on the job and began to feel physically ill from the strain of trying to hold his life together. Thousands of dollars went into counseling that, he says, didn't work. Dozens of evenings were spent in restaurants, considered neutral territory, for more discussions that seemed to go nowhere. Three times Helen packed to leave, and three times Frank convinced her to stay. Finally, they agreed to a permanent split, and Frank moved out, asking for a six-week cease-fire, a stay of events. Within ten days Helen filed for divorce, and within one month Frank contested it.

"You get the feeling you're in a whirlpool that you can't get out of," he explains. "I felt like a character in a soap opera. Here I was, this person whom I considered to be logical doing all these crazy things. Nothing made any sense."

Even when the divorce was final, Frank's problems weren't over. His emotions fluctuated wildly, driving him from despair one day to exhilaration the next. He remains convinced today that the entire procedure was harder for him—in terms of money, in terms of coping with loneliness, in terms of guilt—than it was for his former wife. Finally, Frank went back to the counselors who could not help his marriage but who he hoped could offer him some direction. "I went to find out that I didn't have to be down on myself for the rest of my life because my marriage failed. I went to try and regain some self-respect. I wanted to feel okay again."

In a very real sense, divorce represents death, the demise of a marriage, and it demands, from the survivors, the same grieving process. There is denial, anger and an identity crisis, often more critical for women than for men. The one who initiates the separation has already justified the split; the one who is served notice must grapple with accepting a situation he or she doesn't want. Eventually, however, the divorced person accepts the reality of the separation and begins the process of building a new life.

Divorce is usually the most successful and may even be a desirable option when it is tied to some intrinsic need within one or both of the spouses. The need to escape physical abuse, for example, or the need to fulfill oneself in a legitimate way that the marriage prevents. Classic cases are those of people who have truly outgrown each other and have completely separate life-styles. Nothing holds them together but a legal document that says they are married. Divorce that is based on an extramarital affair tends to be a negative step. So, too, is divorce that is linked not so much to disillusionment with the marriage itself as to disappointment with other areas of one's life, as with the fifty-year-old man who realizes he will never be president of his own company. To compromise for the lost business opportunity, he substitutes a swinging new life-style and the elusive hope of romance.

Frank Riley says he would hope to be married again, and most divorced middle-aged people seem to agree with him. According to the Bureau of the Census, five of every six divorced men over the age of fifty marry a second time; so, too, do three of every four divorced women in the same age group. For them, remarriage has as good or even a better chance than the first marriage.

Approval of friends and family is important to a successful remarriage, but the most critical factor, according to a Florida study, is the level of self-esteem a person brings to the second union. The decision to remarry is a very personal one. If you are divorced and planning to remarry, however, many experts advise waiting for at least one year after the divorce is final. This allows you time to recuperate emotionally, to experience the new you and your new life-style and to know who you are under new circumstances. This also gives time for the patina to wear off any new relationships and lets you see what substance, if any, lies below the surface.

In the final analysis, says Dr. Helm, the individual decides his or her own future and how well he or she will cope with divorce. Frank Riley learned that lesson, and Anne Carson is just becoming aware of it now. Dr. Helm has seen this professionally in her own practice, and, as a woman who has been widowed, and is currently divorced, she has lived the lesson in her own life.

"I know what the personal struggles are," she explains. "And I believe that we are all victims of circumstance and luck in our lives, but that to a large degree it's what we do with our luck, how we perceive it, and how we attempt to adjust our luck that makes the difference. It's the difference between those who lose and those who win."

9

FACING THE SPECIAL PROBLEMS OF WIDOWHOOD AND WIDOWERHOOD

Three of every four wives in this country will become widows, and nearly three of every ten married men will lose a spouse to death over the course of their lifetimes. For women under age seventy-five who are widowed in their first marriage, the median age at widowhood is 50.5 years; this typical widow has one third of her life ahead of her and suddenly she must face it alone. For men, the average age at widowerhood is seventy-one, but nearly one fifth of all widowers are under age sixty.

When their spouses die, these men and women lose, in an instant, an identity that comes from being a partner in a two-person relationship. They encounter immense loneliness today and the prospect of more tomorrow. They struggle with a mix of unfamiliar and often contradictory emotions, and they endure their fate largely alone, living as they do in a society unequipped to offer much more than passing solace. When they might want nothing more than to die themselves, the widowed must cope with the challenge of redefining their lives.

Many factors have an impact on the experience of widowhood. Education, socioeconomic level and the nature of the marital relationship influence the way a person feels when he or she loses a spouse. But, in a very basic sense, the experience is universal. Enough common threads weave through the event that one story contains pieces of many stories and can contribute to a better understanding of the unique problems of being widowed.

"We have to consider being widowed as one of life's crises," says Ida Anger, a Chicago social worker who, through United Charities, conducts education sessions for widowed men and women. "How one accepts the role of being widowed can depend, to a large extent, on the knowledge and understanding one has." Widowhood is a transition that will affect many people, often during the middle years, says Anger. "Learning what one faces in any transition is advisable for everyone."

Marge and Bob Berger had been married twenty-seven years when Bob died, leaving Marge, then fifty-one, alone in the world. The Bergers had been college sweethearts, had married in 1939 and were the parents of two sons. For a short time they lived in New York City. It was an exciting time, says Marge, but after two years they returned to the Midwest to rear their children. Bob became successful in the business world; Marge stayed home with the boys. It was a good life, a busy life. Then it was over.

Today, at sixty-four, Marge Berger works as the registrar of a college of nursing. She is a self-confident and articulate woman, one who has successfully coped with the most traumatic period of her life. She talks now of her memories and struggles, and of her own personal pain and re-engagement into life. She tells her story with the hope that it may help others.

"My husband became ill very suddenly, and we were told he had cancer. After the surgery I thought everything would be fine. I didn't realize that it was a terminal illness. I didn't even let myself think of it when my eldest son flew home on emergency leave from Vietnam. But it all happened very quickly.

"I couldn't believe this had happened to me. Ours was a marriage in which we did everything together. We loved football and went to all the games; we played golf and took vacations together. We enjoyed each other's company. After he died, I used to wait for him to come home. I would stand in the window and watch the other husbands' cars coming down the street. I knew they were going into their houses, where there'd be a family group. Here, I was all alone. It's very hard not to be self-pitying when that happens. It was a very bad time for me.

"My son went back overseas, but the younger one was home with me for a while. He'd missed his exams because he came home when his father became ill, and he was counseled to drop out of school for a semester. It was good for me, because I had someone with me for a while. I had not been one of those helpless wives, however. I had sent out the checks and paid the bills and knew what it cost just to run the house.

"My husband was a fairly young man when he died. He was only fifty-two. We hadn't talked about plans for his retirement or for the future. We were in a very vital time of our lives when everything fell in.

"I tried to think about what had happened. I had no feelings at all and seemed to be in a state of shock. Finally I decided that playing golf, being active in women's groups and taking part in the activities I'd done in the past weren't enough. I felt a great emptiness in my life. I felt I had to get out and get my teeth into something.

"My husband died in February, and in April I took a real estate course. I had a very hard time keeping my mind on what I was doing. The longer I took the course and the more I worked with it, the easier things became. I passed my exam and sold real estate for five years. I later decided that real estate was not my field, but at the time the experience proved invaluable. It got me going again, and for me this was important. My sons both married within four years of Bob's death, and I had no family left, it seemed. I had no one to take up my time. I think when you're in this kind of a situation, keeping busy is the best medicine.

"I used to feel put upon and have a lot of self-pity, even though I realized there were many women in similar situations. I think these feelings have to be worked out individually. I had to find my own answers. I felt my own way and made my own mistakes. I don't think—and this is my opinion—that any widow should make any great decisions for at least two years after the death of a spouse. During the mourning period you don't know what you want. You don't know how you feel. Friends can be kind and caring, but sometimes they can be too helpful and may get angry when you don't follow their suggestions.

"I remember what people said to me. They said, 'Get out of this home. There are too many memories. Go live in an apartment and you won't have these responsibilities. Why don't you take a long trip and forget the whole thing?'

"I feel that running away, on a trip, for example, is not going to help matters. You can't get on a plane and fly away and turn off the fact that you have lost somebody. You can't forget that you will never see him again or hear his voice.

"I also felt that an extended trip was not a good idea at this time because I wanted to maintain a home for both of my boys, until they were on their own. When I finally sold the house, people again tried to tell me what to do. 'Go into an apartment.' But I had lived in an apartment before and didn't want to do so again. I found a smaller, two-bedroom house and moved into that.

"I'm never lonely anymore, though I used to feel overwhelmed by loneliness on the weekends and in the evenings. I have learned over the years not to be lonely. At first you cling to people, your good friends. You become a slight burden because you just can't face time alone. I was never made to feel unwelcomed by my friends, but I finally did realize I would have to learn to make it on my own. I began reading again. I learned to get in my car and go do something. Or I would invite women friends in. I learned that when the cold winter months come, you can put a fire in the fireplace and invite friends over for brunch.

"Now my job keeps me busy. When I get home at night, I welcome the feeling of walking into my quiet home.

"For a while though, I couldn't go places where Bob and I had gone together, and I had a very difficult time for the first couple of years on the anniversary of Bob's death. Now, if the day of his death does not fall on a working day, I plan to be with people.

"Some special days and holidays are difficult too. Wedding anniversaries are hard. Christmas is terrible, because that was always a very special time in our house.

"I've never really considered remarrying, though I have gone out occasionally. If the right person came along, that would be fine. I don't plan to be unhappy, though, if I don't remarry.

"I feel I'm a different person now than when my husband died. I think I'm a stronger person. For so long after Bob's death I was sensitive to what family and friends said or did or didn't do. I hurt so deeply inside that I would look for displays of neglect or abuse from others and in the process made my life miserable. You have to get over that. You must realize that people are too interested in their own lives to inflict pain on others.

"It is important, I feel, as you age, to adapt to change. You must meet challenges and keep busy. I think meeting these goals has helped me through bad times. I do things for myself to keep me interested in life.

"I've told good friends that one never gets over missing someone you've once loved and lost. But with time you learn to handle the feeling."

Medical researchers, psychiatrists and counselors recognize a fairly standard pattern of recovery that normally follows the loss of a loved one. For surviving spouses, the experiences of being widowed are so overwhelmingly strange, they may actually think they are becoming mentally unstable unless they can associate what is happening to them to this larger intellectual model. Surviving spouses need to be reassured that, as unsettling and confusing as their reactions are, they are experiencing normal and appropriate behavior for this type of loss.

In her own education and discussion groups, Ida Anger identifies three stages of loss: First, shock and denial; second, anger and depression or sadness; and third, understanding and acceptance. It is important that the stages be familiar to the person who is living through the grieving process.

During the first period of shock and denial, it is not unusual for widowed persons to feel as if they are standing outside of their own bodies watching themselves going through the motions of the wake and funeral as if they were hosting a party or taking care of the arrangements for a friend. They may even feel that the person being buried is no relation to them or that the entire sequence is nothing more than a bad dream. The deceased is not really gone, they think; he or she will walk in the door tomorrow. This is the time when widowed people often say they feel as if they are losing their hold on sanity.

During the anger and depression stage that follows, the surviving spouse may tend to be irritable with other people for little or no reason. Women often find themselves feeling angry at their deceased husbands—angry because they feel deserted. If the widowed person has a strong religious background, he or she may also feel bitterness toward God and may suffer further from the additional conflict that this causes.

Many widowed persons report a general listlessness and lack of energy during this stage. Friends and relatives may be encouraging them to get out again. But the widowed simply cannot; they are exhausted. If they don't realize that their condition is normal, they may wonder further what is wrong with them.

This is also the time when guilt feelings begin. No matter how objective the circumstances surrounding the spouse's death, some element of guilt on the part of the survivor seems inevitable. This is when he or she begins thinking the doctor was inadequate and the nurses were inattentive and that they personally should have been able to prevent the death from occurring. If a husband dies at home, alone, from a heart attack, his wife may later blame herself: "I shouldn't have been late that day." If a man is killed, accidentally, while crossing the street to his office, his wife may subsequently reprimand herself: "I should have asked him to stay home that day." If a woman dies of cancer, her husband might lament, "I should have known sooner that something was wrong." Ironically, those who had troubled marriages often suffer more during this period than those whose marriages were highly satisfactory. They have more conflicts to resolve. Some may have wished their spouses were gone, and then, when they die, the remaining spouse feels guilty. Some may convince themselves that, given more time, the marriage could have been saved. Before, they always had hope—whether it was real or illusory. Now they have no hope of resolving the old-standing problems. Others may feel the marriage had already begun to improve. Whether this is true or not is hard to say, but that is their perception at the moment. For them, the spouse's death imposes even a greater sense of having been cheated.

In the final stage of grieving, the surviving spouse begins to understand and accept the new situation. "When people reach this point, they are not forgetting their loved one," explains Anger. "Nor are they necessarily happy about their lot. This stage represents the acceptance of the fact that he or she will live the rest of his or her life without this particular mate, a realization that the person can be a whole person again without the spouse." This is the time when people feel free to admit that there are some things —often small things, like staying up late and reading in bed—that they enjoy doing alone, while realizing also that this is not necessarily the life they would have chosen for themselves.

In real life, the stages of recovery are not clear-cut; the edges of one overlap and blur into another. "You will 'hear his footsteps in the hall' for a long time," says Anger, "and this is perfectly normal." There are no timetables that dictate when the widowed should complete one stage and move on to another, although there are some indications that being younger, age fifty as opposed to age seventy, for example, has a positive impact on adaptability. Nor does the recovery process follow a straight upward line; the actual charting of a survivor's progress would in all probability disclose many dips and regressions, some so dramatic that the survivor may feel he or she is back at the starting point, "even though no one ever really is."

In discussions of the widowed state, the question often arises, Who has more difficulty adapting, men or women?

Studies conducted by researchers from the Scripps Foundation of Miami University, Oxford, Ohio, and from the State University of New York at Stony Brook show that factors other than widowhood itself are crucial to an individual's adaptation. Good health, financial security and activities outside of the home appear critical, whether the survivor is a man or a woman. Still, despite the very real difficulties facing the individual widowed man (see page 123, for the experience recounted by one middle-aged widower), women tend, in general, to be at a greater disadvantage, not for any intrinsic reason but because of external factors.

According to preliminary findings in a five-year study at Washington University, Saint Louis, Missouri, widows may face as many as twenty-four different areas of concern or need. These range from loneliness and problems of career and employment to acquiring exact information about their husband's death. Although an individual woman seldom encounters more than ten of these problem areas, says Aaron Rosen, Ph.D., professor of social work and psychology at the university who heads the study, almost inevitably some of the needs she has now are new to her; they are demands that were previously provided for in marriage that must now be met in totally altered living conditions. For example, the widow must cope with financial difficulties; with fears of burglary, rape and physical harm; with problems of house maintenance; with fulfilling her own sexual needs; and with the possibility of arousing negative feelings among her married women friends. In some instances, old relationships go stale because of jealousy; in other cases, the problem is fear. The widowed woman by her very presence reminds the married friend of her own vulnerable position. "People look at me as if I have a contagious disease," one widow said.

Helena Znaniecki Lopata, Ph.D., professor of sociology at Loyola University, Chicago, Illinois, has spent more than a decade studying the problems of widowhood, both in the United States and abroad. Her research reveals that the most overwhelming difficulties facing most widows are economic ones and loneliness. Loneliness comes in many guises.

For example, says Dr. Lopata, a woman may be lonely for the man who has died; she may be lonely for a love object on whom she can focus her attentions; or she may be lonely for someone who treats her as a love object and who considers what she says and does to be important. Some women talk about loneliness for a particular life-style or for an escort or companion. Sometimes women are lonely because their time and work are no longer organized around another person's schedule—breakfast at a certain time, dinner on the table at seven.

Ironically, the women who are best able to deal with widowhood also are the same women most deeply affected by their husband's death, says Dr. Lopata, author of *Widowhood in an American City* and *Women as Widows: Support Systems.* These are women like Marge Berger, women with more education and a more middle-class life-style. This type of woman tends to have had a close relationship with her spouse. While her husband was alive, they were involved in more activities together. They communicated more, identified with each other more, shared more friends, did more parenting together, joined voluntary associations together. When he died, everything he was involved in with her had to be reorganized and restructured.

It is also true that the more education and the more middle-class the life-style, the more personal resources the woman has for rebuilding her life after the period of heavy grief is over. She is often better off financially than is her less educated counterpart. She has self-confidence, her own friends, she knows how to make new friends when the old ones fail her and she knows how to pick up a phone and ask for help if she feels she needs it.

No matter what the personal circumstances of her life, however, the widowed woman eventually must face two major hurdles. First, she must break ties with the deceased, and second, she must do so without feeling guilty. One way she can do this is through what Dr. Lopata calls the sanctification process: The widow idealizes her husband's image and moves him up to sainthood, where he is no longer full of mortal jealousies, so that she is freed of feeling guilt for past problems and for not grieving "enough" as she starts to rebuild her own life. Intrinsic in this second step is the development of a new identity, one that reconstitutes her as a partnerless person.

This period has been found to be a particularly difficult one for widows. They have to get themselves "out of the hole." If they do not face up to the situation, they can become passive for the rest of their lives: They wait for others to come to them; they repeat the same routines everyday; they never make any plans or make any attempt to re-engage or change relationships.

For the traditional woman whose main identity came from the roles of wife and mother, the task of building a new self-image can be overwhelming. "Who am I?" she may ask. This is a valid, agonizing question for many women who are widowed. "Traditionally, the role of the woman has been expressed through the family, by being a good wife or mother," says Dr. Rosen. "Whether this changes in society or not, it does change for the individual once she becomes widowed." Alone now, the widow realizes she has to reach out and initiate the process of redefining her life and of constructing a new way of living. She has to create a new future for herself.

One myth that persists, offered perhaps as reassurance to the widowed woman, concerns remarriage. "Don't worry about anything," women are often told, "you'll get married again." However, according to the National Center for Health Statistics, in one recent year sixty-five of every 1,000 widowed men ages forty-five to sixty-five remarried, compared with fourteen of every 1,000 widowed women in the same age category. Overall, notes the Center, the remarriage rate for widowed men is five times greater than it is for women. Thus, for most widowed women, reality brings a future very different from the kind of past they have known.

The death of a spouse can be a devastating experience. In many instances, the immediate grief affects not only emotional well-being but physiological functioning as well. It can lead to loss of energy, lack of muscular strength, digestive disorders, shortness of breath and tightness in the chest. Often, grieving spouses tend to smoke and drink to excess and to eat improperly. Also, research shows that widowed women tend to take more medications than necessary. To protect their own health and avoid physical harm, recently widowed men and women can benefit from counsel and guidance from their physicians and support from self-help groups of people in similar situations.

Concern for the physical well-being of the surviving spouse is especially important for people in the fifties age group. According to a study at Yale University, as many as half the deaths of widowed persons over the age of fifty can be attributed in some way to the death of the spouse. Men run the greatest risk of failing health within the first six months after the death of their wives. For women, the worst period comes in the second year of widowhood.

A recent study conducted by Knud Helsing, Sc.D., assistant director of the Johns Hopkins Training Center for Public Health Research, Hagerstown, Maryland, compared rates of death and disease among widowed men and women and their married counterparts. Dr. Helsing matched 4,000 widowed persons with 4,000 married persons of the same age, sex and geographic area. By adjusting for risk factors, such as smoking and socioeconomic level, he hoped to pinpoint the exact link between widowhood and mortality.

Dr. Helsing's study solidly substantiates the theory that for men marriage is a healthier state than widowerhood and that for women, in terms of mortality, there is little difference between being married and being widowed. Overall, according to the findings, widowers are 25 percent more likely to die than their married counterparts, and, says Dr. Helsing, there is little doubt that widowerhood itself is a factor in this higher mortality rate. Also, for widowers who remarry, mortality rates, depending on age, are only one-eighth to one-half the mortality rates of widowers who do not remarry.

Over the entire course of the twelve-year study the differences between the mortality rates of widows and their married counterparts and between widows who remarry and those who do not were statistically insignificant. However, Dr. Helsing's data seem to agree with previous reports that mark the second year after the death of the spouse as the most critical for the widow under age sixty-five.

Traditionally, studies have disclosed a link between the widowed person's cause of death and the cause of death of the spouse. "That's not too surprising," says Dr. Helsing, "when you consider the high incidence of communicable diseases and the general lack of sophistication for determining causes of death in the past." Today, he says, such associations are no longer applicable. In fact, with the possible exception of accidents and suicide in the first year after a spouse's death, Dr. Helsing found that causes of death among widowed persons were distributed about the same as among married persons and that there was no statistically significant similarity in causes of death of husbands and wives.

The more than ten million women and almost two million men in this country who have lost spouses can seek assistance from a number of different resources qualified to help them. If you are widowed or know someone whose spouse is deceased, you should learn about the services available in your community. For information, contact your local library, community health center and church or place of worship; you also should look in the telephone directory Yellow Pages under "Social Service Organizations."

In most instances, the widowed must seek out help for themselves. However, some communities have organizations, patterned on Boston's Widow-to-Widow Program, that reach out to the newly widowed man or woman and establish initial contacts. Most of these organizations emphasize the need for peer support. They operate on the premise that only people who have been widowed can truly understand the problems and feelings involved. In fact, studies from both the California School of Professional Psychology and Wichita State University support the value of peer interaction as a critical element in a widowed person's adjustment.

Widowed men and women often feel weak and isolated; they carry emotional loads that they feel they cannot unburden to the rest of the world. Peer groups offer a release from these tensions. The sense of aloneness disappears quickly; the feelings of inadequacy begin to fade as the survivors realize that others suffer also and that not every individual is as strong as he or she may appear.

The heavy weight of emotional trauma is slowly dispersed. "In the rest of society, you can't talk about how miserable you are," says Ida Anger. "In a group session for widowed persons, talking about your feelings is acceptable. It's a legitimate thing to do here."

Although one participant in her classes had been widowed twenty-three years before seeking peer counsel, most people, says Anger, join between eight and thirty months after the spouse's death. Her only caution to widowed individuals: participate in such a group only when you are ready, and come for your own sake, not for anyone else's.

Other vital resources for the widowed are friends and family. In one survey, a Detroit research group found that satisfaction among widowed men and women depended to a large extent on visits from neighbors and on having a confidant or someone to whom they could talk. Those who have a widowed friend can help tremendously by not abandoning the person once the initial flurry related to the funeral is over. "People don't want to listen to me," said one widow. "They 'know' exactly what I need and heap their advice on me rather than wait for me to think and talk it through."

During speeches from city to city, Dr. Lopata is repeatedly asked one question: How can one avoid the pain of grief? "The only answer is to not get married," she explains. "Don't fall in love, because if you love someone, you will be hurt when that person dies. I don't think there is any way of avoiding the pain of grieving. We have to accept it as a normal process of life, as a very tough stage of life. The more people who can help the person talk about it, cry about it, the better."

"Give sorrow words," wrote William Shakespeare. "The grief that does not speak knits up the overwrought heart and bids it break."

PROFILE OF A MIDDLE-AGED WIDOWER

Five months after the death of his wife of thirty-two years, Roger Everett remains in personal limbo. Although the external trappings of his life are unchanged, the central core has become a vacuum. As a widower, Roger Everett struggles to accept his altered marital status. At age fifty-seven, he finds he must choose between living in the past and creating a new identity for himself. To survive alone, he must develop new routines to replace the comfortable habits forged during the years of his marriage. He must also, he has discovered, find new ways of relating to other people and to society.

For Roger Everett, his wife's death did not occur unexpectedly. Late one April, doctors discovered that Nancy Everett had a massive tumor in the lower abdomen. In May—on the Everetts' wedding anniversary—exploratory surgery resulted in a diagnosis of cancer. Despite chemotherapy and radiation treatments, the tumor did not shrink. In November, one month after her youngest son's wedding, Nancy Everett died.

"At first I felt relieved that Nancy's suffering was over," says Roger Everett, a self-employed commodities dealer. "Then the guilt began. I was ashamed of my initial response of relief. I felt terrible that I hadn't visited the hospital on the night she died—it was the last day of her life and I wasn't there. I wondered if I or the doctors could have done more than we did for her, even though, rationally, I accepted the fact that nothing and no one could have altered her fate."

Roger Everett describes his marriage as "more typical than ideal. We had arguments and our various ups and downs," he says. "But we were very close, too. We did many things together." Nine years ago the Everetts moved south, several hundred miles away from their old home and lifelong friends. "That made us even more dependent on each other," says Roger, "But now it leaves me more isolated."

Nancy Everett had been hospitalized for several months before her death. "If anyone was ever prepared for a loved one to die, I guess I was. We knew it was coming and we talked about it openly," says Roger. "The entire period was a rehearsal for the present. But I don't think it [rehearsing for death] really made that much difference. I went through much of my mourning ahead of time, that's all."

Today, Roger Everett's greatest difficulty is in dealing with the loneliness that envelops his life. "In the morning, I wake up to an empty house. In the evening, I have no one to come home to. On the weekends, I am basically all alone and lost."

Roger knows no other widowers. All of his acquaintances and business associates are married. "Whenever I attend a social gathering with them, I feel like excess baggage," he explains. "No one has ever said anything to me, but I sense a bit of animosity from the men whenever I talk to their wives or ask one to join me on the dance floor. I certainly don't think of myself as a threat to their relationships, but maybe they feel differently."

Because he is now alone in the world, Roger feels very strongly that he must make new friends among other unattached people. "But how?" he asks. "I need somewhere to go where I can have rapport with people in my age group, but there are so few places you can meet people. I attended a few meetings of different social groups. I have even had a few dates with widowed women I know, but none of these encounters felt comfortable. I don't intend to be monastic all my life," says Roger, "so sex is a problem, too."

Throughout his marriage, Roger Everett shared household chores with his wife, and he now has hired help come in weekly. But housekeeping still poses a few difficulties. He admits to being baffled by laundry, shopping and cooking chores. "I have no concept of how to plan a week's menu," he explains. "I know *what* you are supposed to do, but I don't know *how* to do it. Most of the time, I exist on TV dinners."

Roger avoids dining out and going to movies, activities he formerly enjoyed, because he feels "foolish" going alone to a restaurant or to a theater. He also hesitates to impose his needs on his married children. One son lives in another state; the other visits him once each week. "They have their own lives," says Roger. "I can't depend on them for my companionship."

For Roger Everett, life has become a series of ritualized routines designed to fill time. "I have taken up a lot more reading," he explains. "I stop for a few drinks with cronies after work or on weekends, something I never did before. I smoke too much. I worry about my job just to have something to think about.

"I am basically an outgoing person, and I have been trying to cheer myself up," he says. "To be honest, however, I would have to say that, emotionally, I am still just limping along."

10

SEXUAL FUNCTIONING AT MID-LIFE

There is a fitness in sexuality at all ages and for both sexes . . .

A Good Age, *Alex Comfort, M.D.*

Sex in mid-life is rarely a clear-cut subject. Many factors influence activity and interest, especially during the fifties, when so many changes seem to occur. Marital status, stress, job shifts and physical health are among the variables that have an impact on one's sexuality. These play against a backdrop of long-standing religious beliefs, social mores and personal preferences. Any meaningful discussion of sexuality must encompass as many of these factors as possible.

At mid-life, it is especially important for you to have correct information about sexual functioning, because sexual functioning changes as you grow older. You need facts on what to expect, on how sex may be different and on how to deal with your continuing sexual needs. It is also possible that, in many instances, we may have acquired incorrect ideas about sex when we were younger; subsequently, we may need to "relearn" some information. "We must appreciate that most of us got our sexual ideas in childhood," says Domeena C. Renshaw, M.D., director of the Sexual Dysfunction Clinic, at Loyola University Medical School, Maywood, Illinois. "We learned in school corridors, from peers little older than ourselves, and we learned, for the most part, erroneous information."

This chapter is concerned with the specific types of factual information most needed by middle-aged men and women. In the first part of the chapter, an interview with an expert husband-and-wife medical team focuses on attitudes and feelings, mythology and reality. Next, the section entitled "Factors That Influence Sexual Functioning" looks at three important topics: Normal physiological changes, problems of dysfunctioning and the nature of the relationship. Finally, a special section presents a selection of the questions most often asked by people in their fifties. These are gleaned from the files of two sex therapists, long-standing leaders in their field.

An Interview with Robert N. Butler, M.D., and Myrna Lewis

Robert N. Butler, M.D., and Myrna Lewis, husband and wife, settle back to talk about sex at mid-life. The subject is a sensitive one to many, but Dr. Butler and Ms. Lewis feel it is an area of concern that must be discussed openly.

Dr. Butler, age fifty-three, former director of the National Institute on Aging, is chairman of the Department of Geriatrics and Adult Development at Mount Sinai School of Medicine, New York. Lewis is a social worker and psychotherapist, with a special interest in women and older adults. They have both dealt with the middle-aged and elderly and have written extensively about the problems and challenges of aging [*Why Survive? Being Old in America,* Butler (Harper and Row, 1975); *Aging and Mental Health* and *Sex After Sixty,* Butler and Lewis (Harper and Row, 1977)].

Their discussion embraces more than just their personal views. Dr. Butler and Lewis are, in a very real sense, speaking for the myriad men and women they have counseled and aided. They speak for dignity and candor, for the right of the middle-aged to live as fully and freely as possible. They believe that sexual activity —like other avenues of human expression—should not be denied because of age.

Dr. Butler, you've been quoted as saying in a discussion on sex and age that mid-life is a time for "gaining skill, confidence and discrimination." Can you elaborate on that for our readers?
BUTLER: By the time you reach middle age, you are more of a person, more of an entity. You have gone beyond the athletic stage of youth and are at a point where you can be more concerned with

the quality rather than the quantity of sex. You can have a real interest in the other person, your partner. That is what skill encompasses, that as you get older you get better at something, if you take it seriously enough.

By this time in life, you have also had some sexual experience and have learned from that experience. This gives you confidence about your abilities. As for discrimination, if you're a middle-aged person, you should be better able to judge your own impulses. You have more of a sense of what to act on and what not to act on. You're better able to judge other people. You can be more sensitive to your partner.

Sex for both of you has the potential to be more fulfilling than ever before—or to be as fulfilling in a different kind of way.

You say different—how can people expect their sexual activities to change as they grow older?
BUTLER: There is no one real answer. Instead, we find a variety of possibilities. On the positive side, there's the potential for perfecting skills that have accrued. There's the possibility of increased good will toward one's partner as well as the likelihood that the two partners will become more comfortable sexually with each other. These factors all contribute to increased pleasure.

On the negative side, you have to consider possible boredom as well as pressure from marital tribulations. These can detract from sexual enjoyment. The reality for most people lies somewhere in between, so we shouldn't look for a single pattern.

Is it more difficult for people to deal with sexual problems in their fifties than at other points in their lives?
BUTLER: The answer to that is *yes* and *no*. No, because people in their fifties often don't think they have all the time in the world for the problem to resolve itself. They may be more willing to wrestle with a problem when it develops. On the other hand, yes, it is harder because men and women at this age may be jumping into something that later might lead to the breakup of a marriage of thirty years standing. From that angle it can be very rough.

You have to remember, though, that if you begin to deal with a problem, you have the possibility of resolution. If you pretend there is no problem, then there is no possibility of resolution.

There are people who by age fifty say they are finished with sex. How do you deal with this attitude?

LEWIS: Everyone has a right to decide what he or she is going to do about sex. The only time you have a problem is when the partner is upset about the decision. Then you have trouble, and the problem needs to be solved.

BUTLER: It is important that people who make this claim look at their motives. Are they genuinely not interested in sex or are they merely living up to a stereotype or to social pressure? There is still a tendency in this country to think that certain activities, and sex is one of them, are for the young—that it is somehow wrong or laughable that older people are interested in and need sexual intimacy.

LEWIS: There are many reasons for denying sexual interest and for giving up sexual activity. The most significant include loyalty to a deceased spouse, some interfering physical problem and religious vows. Others who back away from sex may simply be hiding from other problems. Claiming no interest in sex may be another way of saying they are no longer interested in their spouse. There are probably many women who are simply tired of faking orgasms, who have never really enjoyed sex with their partners and who see this finally as a way out for them. It could also be a way of alleviating anxiety about their ability to function. If there is pain involved, it may be easier to avoid sex than to have the pain diagnosed.

We've all seen the cartoons and heard the jokes—some of them pretty nasty—about sex and age. Overall, do you think this type of comical approach is healthy or detrimental?

BUTLER: People use this type of humor as one way of dealing with their anxieties. The self-ridicule about sex and age—woman as an old hag, man as an impotent being or a dirty old man—helps release some of the tension and worry people have, so in that respect it is good. But the jokes also perpetuate the stereotypes, and that's bad. If you hear them often enough, you start to believe them—they may become self-fulfilling prophecies. People think, "That's what I have to expect as I age," but it's not true at all.

Among the middle-aged, how many ideas and fears relating to sex are bound up in myth or misinformation?

LEWIS: Probably quite a few, affecting mostly the middle class. People on the lower end of the economic scale were too preoccupied keeping things together to worry about such matters. Their concerns were primarily about having too many babies. Intellectuals were well informed as to what was going on, but the middle class was bombarded with erroneous theories and ideas.

For example, up until 1945, the Boy Scout manual warned that if males had sex too often, they would use up their semen and wouldn't have any left for later. If you were a Boy Scout before 1945, you may have believed it then and still believe it now, even though that thinking has been disproved today.

Women especially have to remember the historical period in which they—and their mothers—grew up. Things we can ignore today were very real fears in the 1930s and 1940s, and these were all associated with sexual activity. In the last century, for example, masturbation was thought to be associated with a weakening of the body spirits, which made a person more susceptible to tuberculosis and to mental illness. This idea lingered for a long time. Secondly, venereal disease was not controlled until after World War II. Before 1945, if women caught VD from their husbands—or from lovers—they were branded. It couldn't be cured. They could become sterile. And furthermore their babies could be damaged. This was a very real fear for them. Then there was the terrible problem of unwanted births. For most women, there was no contraception available and no safe or legal way to get abortions. Women faced possible death in childbirth or the possibility of complications after childbirth, to say nothing of the problem of having too many children.

Women who are afraid of sex or who feel negative about sex shouldn't be made to feel humiliated and narrow-minded. They should be helped to put things into perspective and to realize their fears may have been well founded at some point in time.

But how can you reach people and help them think through their beliefs and fears?
BUTLER: I think a conversation like the one we are having now is not a bad idea. People can talk together in a group situation. A person can discuss the matter privately with a physician. Or a husband and wife can talk just to one another. In this way they

will learn about their own and other people's perspectives and views. No one should be heavy-handed and threatening. People should be supportive of the discussion and show respect for different belief systems. If someone has knowledge that permits them to be corrective and supporting, fine; that should be offered, but nothing should be forced on anyone else.

When a husband and wife talk about sex, how can they engage in a conversation without trampling on each other's feelings?
BUTLER: Exposing yourself to such a discussion involves the potential of some short-term bruising to each other's egos. It would be hard to avoid this, but the long-term gain may more than compensate for the initial pain.

If people do not talk at all, there is the danger of becoming estranged and completely avoiding each other sexually. Then the ego can really be hurt. The wife typically thinks, "He doesn't find me attractive anymore." The husband tells himself, "She's not interested in me." I think you have to balance the risks and painfulness of any conversation about sex with the potentially greater risk—the unhappiness, the underlying depression—that can result if you ignore the subject.

Do you find that people who have a strong, active sex life in later years are those who have been sexually active all along?
BUTLER: By and large there is strong evidence to show this, though that doesn't mean that sexual enjoyment can't be developed later in life. It can happen that one who may have had very unsuccessful sexual experiences up to middle age can turn all that around. Generally, however, what we can say about sexual capability is, Use it or lose it.

If you could address yourself to people in their fifties who are interested in maintaining a healthy sex life, what advice would you give them?
BUTLER: If I could say only one thing, it would be this: Look to your physical condition and maintain good health. A lot of the things American men do—especially in regard to drinking—are quite destructive in terms of their sexual activity. The same is true for women, though their problems lie more in the areas of nutrition coupled with physical fitness.

If I could add a second thing, it would be to maintain a good interpersonal relationship with your partner. You have to work at this if you really want to have an interest in sex with your spouse or lover. Don't expect the sexual sparkle to just happen; it is something you have to cultivate.

LEWIS: I feel strongly about three points. First, people don't need to feel embarrassed about their feelings regarding sex. Instead they should develop a respect for where these feelings came from. This will help them sort through where they are now and decide whether they want to stay at a particular point or change. People can change if they want to.

Second, people should learn about medical progress that has been made so that they understand why ideas about such areas as masturbation, impotence and menopause have changed.

And third, using this information, men and women should assume responsibility for their own physical and emotional development as human beings. People can do a lot to improve the quality of life in their middle years if they will use the information that's available and take the responsibility for themselves.

Factors That Influence Sexual Functioning

NORMAL PHYSIOLOGICAL CHANGES AT MID-LIFE

Researchers have found that enjoyment of sex can remain high during the middle years, even though frequency may decline. In some instances, the pleasure that comes from sexual intimacy may even surpass that of the younger years. People may be relieved because pregnancy is no longer possible, and they may feel more relaxed because they have more privacy with the children gone. Many factors can contribute to the personal enjoyment of love-making.

Objectively, however, sex does change. Certain physiological alterations are inevitable in the aging process, and these affect every human activity, including sexual performance. It is important to realize, however, that certain changes are normal, that these biological changes do not reflect on one's masculinity or femininity, and that they do not imply that something is wrong with either oneself or one's partner.

The sexual functioning of women is minimally affected by the aging process. Some women will, in fact, detect increased desire; others will feel little or no difference in their physical response to sexual stimulation. For the majority of women, one or both of the following will occur starting at about age fifty:

• Decrease in or delay of vaginal lubrication.
• A loose, less elastic feeling in the vaginal wall.

For men, more changes are likely to occur than for women. These will affect individual men differently, but some alteration in performance (though not necessarily of enjoyment) is largely inevitable. Normal changes in men include:

• Delayed erections or only partial erections in response to sexual stimuli due to blood vessel and elasticity changes.

• A less acute angle between the erect penis and the abdomen, that is, the erection is not as "high" as before.

• The moment of ejaculatory inevitability may be less well defined. According to William H. Masters, M.D., and Virginia E. Johnson, Sc.D., this "moment" is a subjective sensation that occurs just prior to emission of the male semen. A man actually "feels the ejaculate coming" and at that point has no control over the ejaculatory process.

• The amount of the ejaculate (the semen released by one ejaculation) decreases.

• The force of the ejaculate decreases.

None of these physiological changes makes sex impossible, but they may be distressing if not expected. For couples who wish to remain sexually active, some adjustments may have to be made. These include longer and stronger foreplay, more tactile stimulation (caressing, rubbing and cuddling), finding comfortable positions and use of a lubricating cream. "Basically what we have learned from the people we treat is that sex is worth pursuing despite some obstacles," says Dr. Renshaw. "Only taboos and inhibitions may stand in the way of solutions."

Prior to the 1960s, little scientific data were available about human sexual functioning. Today that is no longer true. Scientific study of human sexuality has documented male and female sex patterns, showing similarities, differences and changes across time. In younger men and women—those below age fifty—the sexual act follows specific, well-defined stages. For the man, for example, the stages are as follows: partial erection, full erection, sustained plateau of erection, point of ejaculatory inevitability, reflex ejaculation and return to pre-excitement phase. For the woman: clitoral swelling, vaginal lubrication and dilatation, sustained plateau of arousal, orgasmic inevitability and reflex orgasmic release.

Starting around age fifty, the stages become less well defined. Lovemaking may progress only partway through the cycle, halt, then be resumed again at stage one at a later time. Almost inevitably, too, more time is needed to complete the full cycle, and this, for the sexually active middle-aged man or woman, may bring a welcomed bonus.

According to Dr. Renshaw, it is important to understand that men between the ages of twenty and fifty go through all six sex stages in an average of 2.8 minutes, whereas women require thirteen minutes to complete their cycle. "Thus there is the classic case of the man rolling over to go to sleep while the woman is left without release of tension." While we blame each other for these problems, it is really the timing difference between the two sexes that is often at fault.

"But this may change after age fifty," she explains, "and most dramatically for men." While on the one hand men find that it may be more difficult to achieve an erection, they may also find that once they have a full erection, they can maintain it for a longer period and thus have a greater chance of satisfying their partner during intercourse. That's why some people say sex gets better as they get older.

It is important that people recognize normal functional changes. They may want to talk about them for reassurance. It is important not to place too much emphasis on coital performance alone. Dr. Renshaw states that, all too often, "making sex" can get in the way of making love. In the long run, rather than bolster sexual satisfaction, a preoccupation with "all or nothing" intercourse can actually detract from true closeness. How two people feel about each other is really the most important ingredient, says Dr. Renshaw, and what you think you can do may be as valuable to you as what you actually can do.

PROBLEMS OF DYSFUNCTION

Problems of sexual dysfunction are frequently encountered in mid-life, but they are not specifically age-related. They can and do affect adults at any age. However, they may also be compounded by the normal physiological changes that accompany aging.

What is important to realize is that in most instances, with proper medical diagnosis and treatment—and with the cooperation and understanding of one's spouse—these difficulties can be resolved satisfactorily.

The following are some of the more common sexual dysfunction problems:

Dyspareunia. This is medically defined as difficult or painful coitus in women. At mid-life, the most common causes of dyspareunia are lack of vaginal lubrication, thinning of the vaginal wall and changes in the shape of the vagina. Artificial lubricants can eliminate the pain for some women. For others, short-term estrogen therapy may be recommended. The hormone can be taken orally or applied locally in specially prescribed creams (see Chapter 7 for further discussion). Regular sexual intercourse itself is recognized as a potential deterrent to dyspareunia.

Physiological response to alcohol and drugs. The use of alcohol, sedatives, narcotics, barbiturates, tranquilizers and certain hypertensive medications can cause physiological reactions that have an adverse effect on sexual behavior in both men and women. Sexual desire as well as performance can be negatively affected.

The effect of alcohol on sexual performance depends on the quantity consumed (as little as 1½ ounces may be critical for some people), individual tolerance (which tends to decrease with age), amount of food in the stomach and the length of time that elapses between the consumption of alcohol and the lovemaking activities.

Drug effects are also linked to dosage, individual tolerance and timing. Any negative effects on sexual performance should be discussed with a physician so that solutions can be sought. In some instances, dosage or timing can be changed or a different drug substituted for the one currently being used. With some drugs, side effects are temporary and will disappear after a few weeks.

Impotence. The term refers to the inability to achieve an erection. Most men are impotent at some time in their lives and for a variety of reasons. Temporary impotence can be caused by illness, fatigue, stress, lack of interest, drugs, alcohol or fear of failure. If a man has occasional difficulty achieving an erection, he is not truly impotent.

Extended impotence. This is defined as the inability to function sexually over a period of months or even years and can have either a psychological or physiological basis or some combination of the two. Psychogenic impotence requires counseling and therapy and is usually most successful when both partners cooperate. Biogenic impotence may be linked to hormonal imbalances that can be tested for and treated (see Chapter 7 for a discussion of the male climacteric) or to any of a variety of other physical problems, such as blood vessel disease, pelvic injury, prostatectomy (surgical removal of the prostate gland), spinal cord injury or diseases of the nervous system. Careful examination and testing can determine whether or not an individual's impotence can be treated.

For some men there is hope in special implants that produce erections by artificial means. In one four-year period at Baylor College of Medicine, Dallas, Texas, 245 men received such devices. The great majority, some 234, reported that they were able to use the implants satisfactorily.

In some instances, potency cannot be returned, but this, says Dr. Renshaw, does not mean that all sexual intimacy and activity must be denied. "There are alternatives to intercourse," she explains. "Caressing, touching and kissing are all means of expressing affection and sexual interest." In one case she treated, the couple's problem stemmed not from the man's impotence—which was physically caused—but from his subsequent total disregard for his wife. "She was in agony not because of his physical symptoms but because he completely shunned her, making her feel rejected as a woman."

It is also important to realize that impotence is not always considered a problem. Some couples are comfortable living without sexual intercourse and adjust to the situation without any difficulty.

Inhibited sexual desire. According to Harold I. Lief, M.D., professor of psychiatry at the University of Pennsylvania School of Medicine, inhibited desire may be the most common sexual difficulty encountered by married couples, but only recently has the problem been recognized as a legitimate sexual dysfunction.

People of all ages are subject to inhibited desire, but it is especially common among the middle-aged. Contributing factors include boredom, lack of variety in lovemaking, loss of interest in one's partner, animosity toward one's spouse and preoccupation with other concerns. Anything that detracts from one's sexual pleasure can eventually contribute to inhibited desire. Thus, depression, feelings of guilt, an inability to perform as well as one would like, preoccupation with traditional stereotypes of the sexless older adults and physical difficulties or illness can also play a role in inhibiting desire.

In dealing with this dysfunction, therapists look for and treat physiological causes, relationship problems and evidence of sexual ennui. "With many people, novelty is an important factor in countering inhibited desire," says Dr. Lief. "We try to get people to enlarge their sexual repertoire, to take long weekends, to get away from the daily pressures. All of these can help reintroduce novelty into their lives."

Dr. Lief cautions that people must be realistic. If people do not love their spouses, if they are having an affair, if they married for money and security, not for love, then virtually nothing can be done to solve their problem of inhibited desire.

Heart disease and diabetes. Coronary disease and diabetes have long been associated with sexual dysfunction in men, but today the thinking has changed or is changing on both counts.

For the most part, there is no biological association between heart disease and sexual dysfunction. Problems tend to be psychological. Women may sometimes think, "If I initiate sex and he has a heart attack, then it's my fault." Men might worry that sexual activity may lead to overexertion. It is not unusual for couples to shy away from lovemaking after a partner suffers a coronary attack, but in most cases sexual avoidance is unnecessary. Although heart rate and blood pressure do rise during intercourse, the increases are equal to those generated by climbing a flight of twenty stairs or participating in other ordinary activities. If a person is tested and found capable of performing varying levels of exercise, he or she will be given the medical go-ahead for having sexual relations. The length of time a person should abstain from sex depends on the type of heart problem encountered and the patient's overall condition.

The connection between diabetes and sexual dysfunction is slightly different, because in some instances the disease can, over a period of time, cause chemically induced impotence. (Generally, however, we tend to associate diabetes with its effects on blood vessels or nerves, or both.) It is not fair to assume that all diabetic men must resign themselves to eventual impotence. In an increasing number of cases, impotent diabetics are being successfully treated, and potency is being returned. "In many cases of impotence, diabetes is only one of many factors involved," explains Dr. Renshaw. "For some men there may be other considerations, and these should be discovered and dealt with."

Dr. Renshaw cites the case of a diabetic, 340-pound, middle-aged man who had used insulin for twenty years and had been impotent for seven years. Discussion revealed that the patient's real sexual problem was psychological. He was haunted by the fear that his teenage children would overhear any lovemaking activities. This, he thought, could cause problems for them, as it had for him when he was growing up. These feelings built up to the point where it was impossible for the man to have an erection. A squeaky bed, not diabetes, was at the base of his impotence. After being advised to place the mattress on the floor for lovemaking sessions, the patient reported his problem solved.

Nonorgasmic response. In a University of Pittsburgh survey of 100 married couples, 15 percent of the female subjects reported an inability to have an orgasm. In addition, 48 percent had "difficulty getting excited," and 46 percent claimed "difficulty reaching orgasm." In large part, these data substantiate previous findings.

A number of factors can contribute to the problem of nonorgasmic response. Physiologically, anatomical differences between partners can help preclude coital orgasm. But even when these problems exist, there is no reason that a woman cannot be helped to climax before or after intercourse.

Psychologically, any inhibitions—disinterest or guilt, for instance—can detract from a woman's enjoyment. "One woman, for example, could not let go sexually because she thought it wasn't 'ladylike,' " says Dr. Lief. "This was an idea she had all these years that stemmed from the way she was reared by her mother and grandmother."

What is important for many women in their fifties and sixties is not so much that they have had difficulty with or never reached orgasm before, but whether they can learn to do so now. The answer that Dr. Renshaw gives is *yes.* Counseling, instruction, permission to explore and understand her own body, as well as more communication with her partner often improves the situation.

Postsurgical problems—mastectomy, hysterectomy, prostatectomy. Neither mastectomy nor hysterectomy have any biological effects that make a woman less feminine or less able to respond to sexual intimacy. Neither operation should preclude sexual activity, after an appropriate recuperative interval, but both can cause attitudinal problems for women and for men. Personal fears and reservations, not the surgery itself, can stifle desire, reinforce misconceptions the partner may have and generally interfere with resumption of normal sexual activities. Because both spouses can have doubts, both should be included in the counseling sessions and discussions that normally take place prior to and following surgery.

Prostatectomy, the removal of an enlarged prostate gland, is fairly common among middle-aged men and, in some instances, can impair sexual functioning. Three techniques for removal are available. The simplest is the transurethral (TUR) technique. It requires no incision; instead the gland is reached and removed by maneuvering a tungsten wire through a tube that is temporarily inserted into the penis. The prostate gland can also be removed using the suprapubic technique, in which an incision is made above the pubic bone and the gland excised. The TUR and the suprapubic techniques rarely result in impotence. The third method is the perineal technique, which requires that an incision be made in the perineum, the area located between the scrotum and the anus. This procedure is the most radical of the three prostate operations and can cause impotence in some men. It must be dealt with on an individual basis.

A common situation following prostate surgery is reversed ejaculation. After the operation, many men no longer ejaculate outwardly. Instead, a climax is reached and semen ejaculates inwardly. It is returned to the bladder and later voided in the urine. There is nothing unusual or alarming about reversed ejaculation. The only problem is that many men confuse the lack of visible ejaculate with impotence. In fact, if they are able to achieve erection and to complete sexual intercourse, they are potent—and they are ejaculating. The process is merely turned around.

Vaginismus. This is an involuntary spasm of the muscles in the lower third of the vagina that precludes penetration by the penis. The condition is treatable and reversible.

Vaginismus may be caused by inflammation or injury. It can also be triggered by anticipation of pain, feelings of guilt or shame or by fear of intercourse. There are no data available on the number of middle-aged women who suffer from vaginismus. Lack of lubrication after age fifty or following a hysterectomy is one common factor that may easily be remedied. When vaginismus occurs, medical assistance should be sought.

THE NATURE OF THE RELATIONSHIP

More often than not, the quality of sex in a marriage reflects the quality of the relationship between husband and wife. When University of Pittsburgh researchers asked men and women to compare their sexual relations with other aspects of their married lives, 63 percent of the women and 60 percent of the men said they were "about the same." When sexual problems develop—especially among the middle-aged—says Dr. Lief, attitudes and difficulties with the relationship are more often the cause than physiological dysfunctioning. "It makes no sense to separate sex from the marriage," he explains. "Sex is really just one important dimension of the relationship."

Stress, boredom and anger are among the factors that can negatively affect sex in the long-term relationship. But there's another side to the story. There are other factors that can, in the long-standing marriage, actually work to make sexual relations strong and healthy.

Researchers have cited eight ingredients considered vital:

- Affection—a sense of genuine concern for the other person.
- Expressivity—the ability to share and be vulnerable, a willingness to be open and honest about feelings and needs, not just those that are sexual but covering all human concerns.
- Sexuality—this is a positive interest in sex, the opposite of inhibited desire.
- Commitment—an honest sense of trust in the other person and a notion of permanency about the relationship.
- Compatibility—having shared interests, at least to a reasonable degree.
- Conflict resolution—the ability to resolve differences and conflicts as they arise without creating overwhelming tension.
- Autonomy—an ability to live alone as well as with one's spouse. This is the opposite of complete dependence.

• Identity—the capacity to feel secure and consistent in one's self-image.

Unfortunately, for many adults, sex remains an anomaly. They can cope well with other problems—child rearing, financial security, family relations—but are devastated by sexual difficulties. A problem with sex often becomes a catastrophe. Worse, it affects not just one but both parties. One may feel inadequate; then the other begins to feel rejected, leading to the "he/she doesn't love me anymore" syndrome.

"In reality, a problem with sex should be treated like any other one of life's difficulties," says Dr. Lief. "A lot of people—probably the vast majority of couples—have sexual difficulties at some point in time.

"Some sexual problems seem to be inevitable, especially in mid-life," he explains. "People should not be completely thrown or taken aback when difficulties arise. No one should feel they are beyond the pale because of sexual problems."

It does, however, take a goodly amount of respect for one's partner to be willing to work out difficulties. As with so much in life, sex is a matter of giving to get.

Sex at Mid-Life: Most Commonly Asked Questions

Many of the questions that middle-aged men and women bring to sex counselors and therapists deal with the physical aspects of sexual functioning. But much of the concern goes beyond the biological. Almost daily, experts are approached about the other aspects of sex—attitudes, mores and specific practices.

We have asked two leading experts on sexuality, Drs. Shirley and Leon Zussman, to share with readers some of the most frequently presented questions. These questions are related to age. They are questions most often asked by men and women in their fifties.

Shirley Zussman, Ph.D., is a practicing psychologist and president of the American Association of Sex Educators, Counselors and Therapists (AASECT).

Leon Zussman, M.D., was an obstetrician-gynecologist on the staff of the Mount Sinai School of Medicine in New York City and a former director of the New York State chapter of AASECT.

The Zussmans, husband and wife, often worked as a team. They are the authors of *Getting Together: A Guide to Sexual Enrichment for Couples* (William Morrow, 1979) and former directors of the Human Sexuality Center of the Long Island Jewish-Hillside Medical Center, New York.

Question asked: "Why am I not as interested in sex as I used to be? Is it age?"

Response: We tell these patients *no,* that their lack of interest does not have to be associated with age. There is no reason that you cannot be active and enjoy sex during the middle and later years. Age may slow the speed at which you become aroused and it may lessen the intensity of the response, but it doesn't mean interest and enjoyment have to disappear. For example, it takes you longer to run around the block and to move about the tennis court than before. Your game is slowed down, but that's no reason you can't continue to play.

Once you deal with the aging myths, lack of interest may still persist. Then the therapists look for other reasons. They try to determine if a couple is avoiding sex because of pain or discomfort or because of conflict—many inner grievances can pile up by the time you are age fifty, and these have to be diminished before sexual interest picks up. Sometimes a wife may say she is not interested in making love when what she is really not interested in is putting up with her husband's behavior. For example, he may sit in front of the television, watch every sports event that is broadcast, then on a minute's notice expect his wife to hop into bed with him. The problem is not that she lacks interest in sex but that she is angry about his neglectful behavior.

Of course, organic factors may play a role in diminishing sexual interest and function, especially in relation to erectile difficulties in men. Every man or woman complaining about a sexual problem in the middle and later years should have a thorough physical examination.

Question asked: "Why does my wife suddenly want more attention from me? She wants to make love more often. She is much more sexual. What's happened to her?"

Response: A number of factors can be intertwined in this type of situation. First, a woman who has remained in the home has no one else to go to for attention once the children are gone. She is more dependent upon her husband now because in a very real sense he is her only close relationship. Second, women who are in their fifties were reared in a time when youth was more inhibited than in today's world. These women have grown older, and their inhibitions have sometimes broken down. They see evidence all around of the "sexual revolution," and with the children gone they feel freer. Suddenly, they begin thinking, Why not? I don't want to have missed this.

A third reason is linked to one's perception of self. The fifty-year-old woman may feel she is not as attractive as she once was. To combat this, she needs physical intimacy and the reassurance lovemaking brings.

The need for more attention is not always manifested by the wife, however. Men may also experience many of the anxieties tied to loneliness and a diminishing sense of self-worth. Then they too make increased sexual demands on their spouses. The problem in many marriages is that both partners are not at the same point at the same time. Communication is essential to help them understand where each one is and to help bring them closer together.

Question asked: "Does lovemaking always have to end in intercourse?"

Response: We tell people the answer is no. In fact, in many cultures, people feel free to show affection without being pressured into having sex. Unfortunately, our tradition is not like that. We grow up thinking that love play must end in intercourse. Sex really involves a broad panorama of experiences, and people have to be told this. They also have to learn to communicate their feelings to each other.

For example, a man approaches his wife and she shuns him. Maybe she would like to be caressed and touched but she thinks he wants to have intercourse, which she isn't in the mood for right now. Instead of saying "Yes, but," she says "No." Then she comes to us and asks, "Why does my husband always want intercourse every time he touches me?" We ask him, and his response is "Well, doesn't *she* always want intercourse when I touch her?"

Or you have the man who complains that his wife isn't interested in making love. We ask her the reason, and she says she *is* interested—but all he wants is penetration; she wants to be held and fondled. They have different definitions of what lovemaking is.

We advise people not to try to be mind readers. You just cannot do it. You can tell someone how you feel and ask how he or she feels, but you cannot assume anything. You must always ask. You must say, "I feel this way, how do you feel?"

When people realize they don't have to have a goal every time they feel like being close and tender with each other, they feel much more relaxed. We have had men end up admitting great relief at not having to have intercourse every time they become affectionate. "I can touch and caress, even bring my wife to orgasm, and I don't have to have an erection that night," one man said.

Question asked: "Is masturbation normal?"
Response: This question comes up constantly and continually. We define *normal* as any activity that does not offend, does not hurt, does not cause discomfort and is enjoyed by a couple. We try to do away with some of the old myths and to reassure both men and women that masturbation does not have any psychological or physiological aftereffects. It is amazing, however, how many people associate a sexual problem with masturbation. We have had men ask if their current potency problems stem from the fact that they masturbated too often when they were younger. There are still many people who have doubts about masturbation. We tell them that rather than being harmful, from a biological standpoint, it is very useful in maintaining the physiological reaction of arousal and climax. Psychologically, it often restores a sense of well-being and satisfaction when a partner is not available or the mood is to satisfy oneself.

Question asked: "How often should we make love? What is the 'right' amount for people our age?"
Response: There is no right answer. Normal and right is whatever you are comfortable with.

If one couple is happy having intercourse once a year, that is completely normal. If another couple is happy having intercourse every night, that is completely normal. But if one of the partners wants to make love once a year and the other wants to do so nightly, then that couple has a problem. The challenge is to reach a compromise that is acceptable to both.

As with so much involved with sex, it is not a matter of one person being right and the other person being wrong. Rather, it's a matter of compromise, of finding what is agreeable to and enjoyable for both parties.

11

EXERCISE AND SPORTS IN MID-LIFE

Even at a distance, Frank Sedgman looks like an athlete. He has the swift, easy gait; the lean, hard strength; and the confidence of a winner. And that he is. In 1952, only one year after winning the United States singles title in tennis at Forest Hills (the first Australian to do so), Sedgman captured the coveted crown at Wimbledon. Twenty-eight years later, Sedgman continues playing to applause and racking up victories in the tennis Grand Masters circuit (a touring group of past international tennis champions). In fact, at age fifty-two, the gentleman from "down under" is acknowledged as one of the best tennis players in his age group in the world.

If it hadn't been for the Grand Masters, says Sedgman, he would have been a lost resource long ago. "The tournaments have literally brought me from the scrap heap back onto the courts."

How does it feel?

Sedgman flashes a smile. His deep-set blue eyes survey the waiting courts at the Country Club of North Carolina, Pinehurst, where he will begin competing again in two days. "Pretty good," he says quietly in British-inflected speech. "It's nice to know you can still play a good game of tennis."

When the Grand Masters circuit first began in 1973, Frank Sedgman had some doubts—not about his ability to play but about audience reaction. "I really didn't think the idea of older players would catch on, and I wondered why people did come to watch. Did they think we were just a bunch of freaks, or were they there to enjoy good tennis?" Today, he has his answer. "We are accepted the world over for what we are," he explains, "middle-aged men in pretty good shape who can put on an interesting and competitive tennis match."

As players grow older, the type of game they play naturally changes. Sedgman is not as fast as he was in the earlier days, his serve is not as powerful, nor is his grip as strong. "But you make trade-offs," says the champion. "You play a better defensive game. You are more patient and wait for the other person to make mistakes. You're steadier on the ground strokes."

Sedgman claims he works as hard now at keeping fit as he ever did, but, again, he has had to make some adjustments. "I do more stretching to keep flexible and help prevent tearing a muscle, and I ration my energy carefully. You have a set amount of vitality. You have to find a happy medium." Sedgman learned his lesson the hard way in 1968, when he overtrained for an open tennis tournament and subsequently had to drop out because of "tennis elbow."

"I tried to train the way I had twenty years ago. I thought I could do it. It was a painful lesson to discover that I couldn't."

To keep in shape, Sedgman runs three or four miles a day, a practice he started as a teenager. He also plays squash and golf several times a week. On tour, he plays as much as four hours of tennis the day before a tournament begins. "I still end up feeling stiff and tired the day afterward," he explains, "but I accept this as part of the game."

Frank Sedgman learned to play tennis during the Depression. His father, a carpenter, was often unemployed, and as a young boy Sedgman often came home from school to find his parents out on the public tennis courts. "I used to watch and sometimes play with my father, but it wasn't until I began winning a few tournaments in school that I became really interested. Winning was my reinforcement.

Sedgman continues to enjoy rewards from playing the game he loves. Money is one incentive. In one recent year, he earned nearly $100,000 on the Grand Masters tour. But even more important to him is that thrill of winning. "You get elated just the same as when you were younger," he explains. "When I can't win anymore, that's when I will think about quitting."

For Frank Sedgman, tennis provides a sense of physical well-being, a feeling of control over self and an ego-boosting respect from admirers. "Because of the Grand Masters circuit I am still legitimate as a tennis expert. People can still talk to me as someone who is competing on a fairly high level, not just as a champion of a bygone era."

Important also is the satisfaction that comes from having set a precedent. "Sure there is a sense of nostalgia to all this, but I don't really like to talk about the old days too much," he says. "I would rather live in the present. I like what I am doing now. I believe in taking life as it comes. There is nothing I can do about getting older except to make the best of it and get as much out of it as I can.

"We are doing what has not been done before—on a grand scale. We are opening horizons for younger people, giving them something to anticipate later on, and we are showing people our age that it is worthwhile to maintain physical activity. Look at the lot of us. We make a good case for the argument that if you keep up your conditioning, you can retain your vitality.

"It's especially sweet in light of the fact that a decade ago I never would have dreamed this would be happening. I suppose," he admits modestly, "that you could say we're a bit of an inspiration."

From tennis and golf, to swimming, skating, bicycling, running and rowing, regular exercise for men and women in their fifties —and sometimes competition in sports—is catching on.

"The stereotype of aging says it is impossible for people to do certain things when they grow older, that it is impossible to do better today what we did yesterday," says Alex Ratelle, M.D., age fifty-six, senior consultant and former head of the anesthesiology department at Methodist Hospital, St. Louis Park, Minnesota. "But there are too many people out there proving the stereotypes wrong." Dr. Ratelle should know.

Fifteen years ago, when he began jogging through his Minnesota community, Dr. Ratelle was the object of public ridicule. "I was sweating, and people weren't supposed to sweat if they could avoid it," he explains. "I was a crazy guy running around in my underwear."

At the 1978 Chicago marathon, two policemen physically removed Dr. Ratelle from the front row—a spot he had earned— and forced him further back into the pack. "Some of my friends were teasing me about being up front and kiddingly told the police to get the old man out of the way. The two officers took one look at my gray hair and decided I didn't belong up there." But the laugh is on them, he explains, and on all those who for years believed that if you were middle-aged, you were over the hill in any physical sense of the word.

At this writing, Dr. Ratelle holds four world records for his age. Just recently he completed his best marathon time in three years. Unfortunately, however, most middle-aged adults do very little in the way of physical exercise. According to a recent Gallup poll, 47 percent of the American people claim to take part in daily physical activity, but most of those who actually do are the young and the better educated. The President's Council on Physical Fitness and Sports says that, despite inflated figures to the contrary, less than half the adult population in this country exercises regularly, and less than one-third participate in any sports activities at all.

In part, this widespread inactivity stems from the mythology that surrounds the issues of exercise and aging. As people grow older, they tend to believe that their need for physical activity diminishes and they tend to exaggerate the risks involved in vigorous exercise after middle age. They also underrate their own physical abilities and capacities while overrating the benefits of light, sporadic activity. As a consequence, they then do nothing physically taxing on any regular basis.

Dorothy and Harry Stoner are exceptions to the rule. Dorothy, at age fifty-six, rides an exercise bicycle daily for fifteen minutes, walks to and from bus stops on her way to work and plays tennis. Harry, fifty-seven, runs five miles every morning. Last year the couple took up cross-country skiing, and this year they joined a church bowling league. Among their circle of twenty largely middle-class friends and acquaintances—all of whom are in their fifties—Dorothy and Harry are the only active pair.

"Although the others admire Harry for running, they basically think we are both crazy," says Dorothy. "Their attitude is one of 'Why bother?' When you mention doing something physically taxing, they have nothing but excuses—too tired, not enough time. Their response to an invitation to go cross-country skiing was 'We'll break our necks!' So they sat in front of their televisions while we went out and had a great time."

Sitting, says Dorothy, is what her friends do more of than anything else. During the day they work at sedentary jobs; in the evening they delight in two or three drinks while resting from their jobs. On weekends they watch television, play cards, go to dinner together and visit. "I honestly don't know what it would take to get them moving," says Dorothy. "Nothing we have said has made any difference."

"The biggest problem for most middle-aged adults," says Charles T. Kuntzleman, Ed.D., national program consultant to the YMCA, "is that they hate exercise, not in and of itself, but because of past associations and ideas."

As teenagers, today's fifty-year-old women were told that exercise and sports would make them appear masculine. The message went like this: You are grown up now, stop acting like a tomboy. As a consequence, many women never learned a physical activity they could enjoy. They still feel it is somehow unladylike to be physically active. Even if they want to try something, they often feel incompetent and threatened.

For men, the word *exercise* conjures up images of a gym teacher or army sergeant yelling at them. The memory that men have is that exercise is somehow punitive. Those who participated in sports activities at least enjoyed some immediate rewards for their efforts, but, even for most of them, involvement ceased years ago. Today these men think of sports in terms of television viewing, not in terms of their own participation.

If you are a viewer rather than a participant, you must first come to terms with these psychological barriers if you are to become active in sports or regular exercise in mid-life. You must understand your own fears and then plot a sensible course of action for dealing with them.

"I know how difficult it is to get started—I've been there," says Dr. Ratelle. "But it is really something you owe yourself. Right now you are at a crossroads in your life. You can literally decide on the kind of life you want to lead, whether it will be active and adventurous or inactive and dull. You can decide on the type of person you want to be, either one lost in indulgence, trying to find fulfillment in an increasingly complicated and sophisticated world, or one who has returned to the simpler pleasures of your younger years.

"Being physically active can change your self-image. It can give the feeling of satisfaction and achievement that many of us have lost along the way. It can give you goals and challenges for your future. There are no guarantees, but through exercise you can create an insurance policy that promises a stimulating life and the opportunity to enjoy it."

Fitness and Health

"Active people have already passed the real-life stress test," says Dr. Ratelle. "Their metabolic and organ systems have already demonstrated that they can handle stress. The active person probably has practiced good nutrition, probably doesn't smoke, probably consumes smaller quantities of alcohol than a nonactive counterpart and, by and large, has a lower body fat content. You're dealing with a stronger system to begin with."

Scientists still have no proof that exercise and physical activity can actually prolong life, but they are accumulating data that link physical fitness to improved quality of life. In fact, the National Institutes of Health says exercise may be "the most effective anti-aging pill ever discovered."

Exercise is valuable on two counts: First, it *trains* the body. Training implies a honing of skill, making the most of what the body has to offer. It improves bodily functions and decreases the chance of malfunctioning. Second, exercise can act in a *healing* capacity. That is, in some instances, it can help correct physiological illness. Following is a summary of the available knowledge concerning exercise and its impact on the human body.

Training Aspects of Exercise

THE CARDIOVASCULAR SYSTEM

Research shows that exercise affects the entire cardiovascular system. Regular physical activity produces positive changes in the blood, the blood vessels and the heart.

Blood. Exercise increases the number of red blood cells in the body, and this helps to increase the oxygen supply to the body's muscles. This is important because the more oxygen available to the muscles, the more efficiently and effortlessly the muscles can function.

Exercise also slows the rate at which lactic acid is formed. Lactic acid is a waste product of active muscles; when it overflows into the bloodstream, it inhibits movement and can lead to cramps. The less lactic-acid buildup, the easier it is for you to be active.

Activity produces other important changes in the blood. Recent studies show that exercise lowers levels of low-density lipoprotein (LDL) cholesterol, the type of cholesterol often associated with incidents of heart disease, and increases levels of high-density lipoprotein (HDL) cholesterol, a type of blood protein recognized as a deterrent to heart disease. Researchers also link exercise to a drop in triglyceride levels, other blood fats linked to the development of atherosclerosis and stroke.

Exercise can even help prevent blood clots. In a study at Duke University Medical Center, Durham, North Carolina, sixty-nine adults, aged twenty-five to sixty-eight, participated in a ten-week conditioning program. Testing showed that exercise (ten minutes of stretching and thirty to forty-five minutes of walking, three times a week) helped fight blood clot formation by increasing plasminogen activators, proteins that dissolve other clot-forming components. This is important because, if a clot occurs, the faster it is dissolved, the better the chance that serious medical consequences from any blockage will not occur.

Still under investigation at the center is the effect of exercise on platelets. These are blood corpuscles implicated in the development of atherosclerosis, heart attack and stroke. "We have evidence that being physically fit affects the way platelets function," explains Duke University cardiologist R. Sanders Williams, M.D., "but our data are preliminary, and we can't be certain of the clinical significance of this finding yet."

Blood vessels. To function properly, the heart needs an ample supply of blood, and exercise can increase the heart's blood supply in a number of ways.

First, exercise can enlarge the diameter of the main coronary arteries. The wider the arteries, the more easily blood flows through them.

Second, as mentioned previously, exercise helps reduce the concentration of fat in the blood. Fatty deposits can clog arteries and inhibit blood flow. Low levels of fat deposits result in increased blood flow.

Third, exercise increases the number of blood vessels that serve the heart muscle. This results in an overall increased supply of blood throughout the entire heart. It is believed that the auxiliary blood vessels developed as a result of exercise can supply needed blood to portions of the heart that might be deprived of blood because of thrombosis (blood clot) or atherosclerosis (buildup of fatty substance and narrowing within an artery) of the coronary arteries, conditions that can result in heart attack.

Exercise also increases the number of blood vessels in skeletal muscles. This means that, as a result of physical conditioning, more blood and the oxygen it transports are made available to working muscles. The overall result is improvement in general functioning.

Heart. The aging process has two basic effects on the heart.

First, it tends to reduce the heart rate. The maximum heart rate that can be attained in young adults is 200 beats per minute; in persons approaching age sixty, the maximum rate is 160 beats per minute or less.

Second, aging also reduces cardiac output and stroke volume, the amount of blood the heart pumps with each beat. The heart muscle becomes weaker and less efficient. The annual loss of muscle strength after age twenty is approximately .85 percent.

Exercise is valuable because it tends to minimize these age-related changes in the heart. Exercise has been shown both to increase maximum attainable heart rate and to improve cardiac output and stroke volume. Conditioning also helps the heart develop an important reserve capacity, that may be vital in any stressful situation.

But even when no work is being done and the body is resting, physically fit people have an advantage. Their hearts can beat at a reduced rate and still keep the body supplied with all the blood it requires. In most individuals the "normal" resting heart rate is 72 beats per minute. In the conditioned individual, it can drop as low as 40 beats per minute. Thus even at rest the trained heart works only half as hard as the untrained heart.

Many of the cardiovascular changes brought about by exercise are measurable only in sophisticated scientific laboratories, but some can be felt directly by individuals who exercise. "You will feel stronger," says Dr. Williams. "You will be able to climb with less effort." The problem is that people expect immediate changes. When they don't notice an improvement in two or three weeks, they give up.

"We have found in our subjects that it takes about six to ten weeks before people notice any difference," explains Dr. Williams. "But it only takes two or three weeks to lose the benefits once you stop exercising."

THE PULMONARY SYSTEM

Exercise has little direct effect on the pulmonary system. But it has an overall indirect impact on the respiratory process that is critical to optimum functioning.

The lungs have no muscles of their own. The amount of air you are able to take in with each breath depends upon the diaphragm muscles, the abdominal wall and the muscles between the ribs. By strengthening these muscles, exercise can affect lung expansion and can thus increase your body's supply of air.

At rest, an average man inhales approximately 6 to 8 liters of air per minute. During a period of maximum exertion, the same man may take in 100 liters of air per minute. The more air an individual takes in, the more oxygen is made available to the body. However, the rate at which an individual can extract oxygen from the air supply depends on the number of red blood cells in the blood and on the speed and efficiency with which the heart moves the body's blood supply through the lungs. Thus, how well the pulmonary system functions depends directly upon the cardiovascular system. Through its direct effects on the cardiovascular system, exercise exerts an indirect but crucial influence on the pulmonary system.

The maximum amount of oxygen an individual can extract from the body's air supply and deliver to the muscles is called V_{O_2} MAX (V = volume; O_2 = oxygen; and MAX = maximum). V_{O_2} MAX, which is largely determined by your genetic makeup, tends to decline with age. Exercise, however, can help halt or even reverse this decline. According to a Swedish study, a few months of vigorous physical work can increase V_{O_2}MAX by as much as 15 to 20 percent.

We equate vitality or personal energy with the amount of physical activity we can accomplish. Our activity level is directly linked to the amount of oxygen available to the body's muscle system, which, in turn, depends upon both the cardiovascular and the pulmonary systems. Because exercise affects the two systems that control the body's supply of oxygen, a regular program of exercise plays a critical role in determining how much vitality you will enjoy in your middle and later years.

THE MUSCULOSKELETAL SYSTEM

The human body contains some 200 bones and 600 different muscles, all of which benefit to some extent from exercise. The primary impact of regular exercise on the skeletal system can be the prevention of osteoporosis, bone loss associated with mid and later life, especially in women (see Chapter 7 for a discussion of osteoporosis).

The effects of exercise on muscles are more extensive. With exercise, both muscle enzymes and mitochondria, cellular energy producers, increase and become more active, converting more fats and carbohydrates into energy for the body to use. Physical activity also causes muscular contractions, which thicken muscle fiber and increase the number of connective tissues within the muscles. This strengthens muscles. It is important to remember that muscles are made to be used. They don't wear out because of activity. In fact, the opposite is true. When muscles are not used, they lose strength and eventually atrophy.

Exercise combats muscle stiffness, which usually crops up during mid-life, even among active adults. Stiffness is caused by chemical linkages, or side chains, that develop around muscle tissue. When you are young, you don't notice them because you're growing constantly, and you automatically break the side chains. But when you stop growing, there is nothing short of exercise to break the linkages.

You don't have to be inactive for long periods to feel the effects of the linkages. They literally develop overnight and can make you feel stiff in the morning. The best antidote is simple stretching.

When you break the chemical linkages that cause stiffness, you also help your joints function properly. This is important. When a joint is used properly and moves through its full range of motion, physical stress is shared equally over the entire cartilage area of the joint. Limited joint action, which can result from strong muscle side chains, places undue stress on only part of the cartilage and causes that area to erode more quickly than normal.

If you have had knee cartilage removed, you should avoid any unnecessary use of and stress on the knee joints. Jogging and skiing are not recommended. Instead try swimming, which decreases the pull of gravity and eliminates stress from the knee area.

WEIGHT CONTROL

Exercise can help you lose and control body weight not simply because it uses up excess calories stored in the body, but rather because of its method of doing so. When you diet, you lose both fat and muscle tissue. When you exercise, however, most weight loss stems from a decrease in body fat. Rather than depleting important muscle tissue, you're actually building it up. The more muscle tissue you have, the easier it is for you to be active, and the more active you are, the less you'll gain excess weight.

While short bursts of exercise may increase appetite, extended periods of activity actually help stabilize your desire for food, another benefit for those trying to lose weight. Any dramatic drop in blood sugar will make you feel hungry; but during prolonged activity your body doesn't draw upon this sugar as an energy source. Instead it uses body fat, leaving the sugar level relatively stable.

Exercise also speeds up the rate at which food moves through the intestinal tract, giving the body less time to convert food supplies into fat. And it increases the metabolic rate, or the speed at which food is utilized. An efficient, trained metabolism keeps working at a higher speed for five or six hours after an exercise session is complete.

To lose weight through exercise, you must use more calories than you consume. Generally, you need ten to fifteen minutes of vigorous exercise per day to use up 100 excess calories. Walking just one extra mile every day can mean losing ten pounds in one year.

Healing Aspects of Exercise

MENTAL HEALTH

In a University of Wisconsin, Madison, study of a group of mildly and moderately depressed patients, an exercise program involving activity three times a week helped more than half the subjects feel better without antidepressive drugs. In response to a University of Illinois, Chicago, questionnaire, 2,500 adults who claimed to exercise regularly said that physical activity helped reduce feelings of tension. A study at the University of Pittsburgh (Pennsylvania) associated vigorous exercise with a decrease in anxiety levels among sixteen male subjects.

No one knows exactly how physical activity affects the mental state, but several different theories are available. Exercise increases the flow of oxygen to the brain, and some researchers say this accounts for an improved sense of well-being. Activity is also linked to a decrease in body salts, which, in some instances, have been associated with mental depression. Exercise promotes deeper sleep in many people, and this may lead to a more positive mental attitude. It is also possible that exercise increases the amount of the hormone norepinephrine in the brain. Low levels of norepinephrine are associated with depression, while high levels are found in people who describe themselves as feeling happy and positive.

DIABETES

Diabetes mellitus, the disease that tends to afflict young children, stems from an inability of the pancreas to produce insulin. Adult-onset diabetes, which usually appears during mid-life, is caused not by the body's inability to manufacture insulin (the pancreas, in fact, usually produces a normal amount of the hormone) but by its inability to use the insulin that is available.

Exercise helps counter diabetes because it stimulates the growth of cell-surface receptors for insulin, and with more receptors the cells are better able to use the insulin that the body produces. For some victims of adult-onset diabetes, exercise can virtually reverse the condition and eliminate the need for any medication.

HEART DISEASE

Although all cardiologists do not agree that exercise is beneficial in the rehabilitation of heart disease victims, current thinking seems to be moving in that direction. Physical activity was once considered harmful to the damaged heart. Now, thanks to better research techniques, scientists know that exercise provides the same beneficial effects for the heart attack victim as it does for the person without heart disease. It may take longer for the heart patient to realize the benefits of exercise, but in the end, he or she is better protected against future cardiovascular problems.

Five years ago, heart attack victims were generally hospitalized for three weeks, then kept out of work for six months or longer and finally cautioned to restrict their activities for the remainder of their lives. Today, it is not unusual for a heart patient to be released from the hospital in seven to ten days, to be back at work, at least part-time, in six to eight weeks and finally to be encouraged to get going again, usually through some type of exercise program. "We know today that we can take people who lead restricted, almost invalidlike existences because of heart disease and, through physical conditioning, greatly expand what they can do," says Dr. Williams.

However, he admits that this return to nonpharmacologic ways of treating heart disease is contrary to the trend that medicine has taken and that people have come to expect. "We are advocating low technology in a highly technological field. We are telling people they have to do the work."

HIGH BLOOD PRESSURE

Research shows that regular exercise can help lower blood pressure in individuals suffering from hypertension or high blood pressure. In some instances the drop is substantial. In others it is slight, but in the majority of hypertensive individuals who exercise, some decrease does occur.

Blood pressure is the force that is exerted against arterial walls as blood is pumped from the heart and moved through the elaborate array of vessels that extend throughout the body. *Systolic* pressure is the pressure exerted on arterial walls when the heart is working, that is, when it is pumping blood into the system. *Diastolic* pressure is the pressure exerted on arterial walls when the heart is between beats. When a blood pressure measurement is taken, the systolic pressure is given first, and the diastolic pressure is given second.

High blood pressure can be caused by a number of factors, including stress, excess weight and a genetic tendency toward the condition. The exact mechanism by which exercise lowers blood pressure levels is not clear. In some instances, it is thought that exercise reduces elevated blood pressure by contributing to weight loss or to the reduction of tension. It is also possible, in some cases, that blood pressure is lowered because of exercise-related changes in the cardiovascular system. As mentioned previously, exercise can reduce levels of cholesterol and other fatty deposits and it can help enlarge the diameter of the main arteries. These changes, in turn, can lessen resistance to blood flow and thus reduce the amount of pressure or force needed to move blood through the body's blood vessels.

One word of caution is necessary: When we talk about exercise having a beneficial effect on high blood pressure, we are referring to the long-range benefits of a regular program of physical activity. During actual periods of physical exertion, systolic pressure rises in most individuals. (People whose blood pressure does *not* rise during exercise are at a high risk.) Therefore, it is important that men and women who have high blood pressure (and those who do not but are in middle age) check first with their physicians before beginning any exercise program.

ARTHRITIS

Exercise does not cure arthritis, but it can help the arthritic victim preserve a full range of movement and maintain a positive mental attitude. Paula Robertson is a case in point.

Fourteen times each week, Paula Robertson climbs onto a 4-x-6-foot wooden platform at a local community center, turns on a cassette tape of specially selected music, shouts, "Let's go," and begins leading eighty to a hundred men and women of different ages, shapes and abilities through forty minutes of total body movement. The workout is rigorous. "You should be sweating," Paula says after ten minutes of warm-up. "Don't stop. Never stop," she calls out halfway into the session. And every minute, it seems, she is smiling and setting an example for her students.

"People don't realize," Paula explains, "but every time I get up on that table, it hurts—until I get moving. Then comes the feeling of freedom, the incredible joy that comes from being able to move."

At age fifty-two, Paula looks the picture of health. She stands tall and erect. Her eyes are quick, and her blond hair is perfectly coiffed. She has the figure and movements of a professional model —which she was some thirty years ago. She has the natural presence of one who works easily with the public, and this too she has done for nearly three decades. What she does not resemble, leading her class through an exercise session, is a victim of severe arthritis, which she is. Her disguise, her ability to outwit the disease that had crippled her for an entire year, and that today still threatens, Paula credits to exercise.

"I don't think it's an exaggeration at all to say that exercise has kept me alive," she says. "I know this is true."

Paula was twenty-two years old when arthritis struck. At first she noticed only minor aches and pains, but within months she was virtually disabled. The disease forced Paula, then a college sophomore, to drop out of school. The pain forced her to walk in a slump—or not to walk at all. "I remember standing in the kitchen holding onto the sink unable to move because it hurt so much, and I remember my father having to carry me to the car."

The only time Paula was able to function normally was when she was taking massive doses of medication—tranquilizers, muscle relaxers and as many as thirty aspirin a day. For an interim, at least, she was able to return to a regular routine. She began taking modeling assignments, both as a source of income and to fill her time. She also began thinking of her future.

"More than once I was told to prepare for life in a wheelchair. 'You'll just have to learn to live with this.' That was what everyone said. Well, I didn't want to live like that," she explains. "Finally I realized that, in the end, despite the sympathy and concern that everyone had for me, this was something I would have to face alone—so I rebelled."

Paula wanted to be active again. The former dancer and former swim-team captain had too many memories of how good her life had been when she was moving about and active. "I wanted to be my old self again."

"Is there ever a time you feel good?" a physician once asked Paula.

"Yes," she said. "When I'm moving."

"Then move as much as you can," he directed. And for thirty years, she has followed that advice.

First, Paula went back to school, this time majoring in physical education. Next she volunteered to teach swimming for the Red Cross and took a night job coordinating activities at a local community center. The more active she was, Paula discovered, the less pain she experienced and the more freely she could move. Eventually she dropped all medication, except for an occasional aspirin, and developed a philosophy and mode of life that kept her moving. She is today a full-time professional exercise consultant and she has never forgotten to what she owes her own vitality.

One day a fifty-year-old former professional football player came to her exercise class, on a dare from his wife. "This will be nothing, a piece of cake," he told Paula beforehand. "I play tennis and touch football. I swim. Your class will be a cinch." But it wasn't. After the session the man returned to the podium, humbled. "I can't believe how out of shape I really am," he admitted.

"Men need push-ups and sit-ups," another male participant once challenged. "This isn't the right kind of class." Paula looked at the man, asked him to do a few simple flexing movements and when he could not, suggested that he give the class a two-week trial. Several years later, the man continues attending the class.

A fifty-four-year-old woman in one corner of the room groans her way through some of the more vigorous twists and turns. "Don't get me wrong," she says, "I'm not complaining. Four years ago I couldn't move at all. I couldn't lift a fork. I have arthritis. I love this class."

When she doesn't exercise, says Paula, she suffers the consequences. "Seventy-two hours into a vacation without my classes and I can't bend; in the morning I can't straighten up. I walk holding onto the edges of tables and the backs of chairs."

Will she ever stop?

"I can't envision that. I might slow the pace or focus for a select age group, but stop exercising altogether, no," she says. "I can't. I *have* to keep going."

Getting Started

Which exercise is best for you?

• Dr. Ratelle, M.D., the anesthesiologist and champion runner, advocates running, not only for its physiological benefits but for the psychological sense of purpose and well-being it promotes. But if you can't run or you don't want to, he suggests walking or the use of an exercise bicycle.

• Dr. Williams, M.D., the cardiologist, recommends that you try a combination walk-run program tied to overall life-style changes that incorporates more activity into your daily routine.

• Dr. Kuntzleman, Ed.D., YMCA exercise consultant, suggests that you try walking, because it requires no special skill and because it will reintroduce you to the pleasures of being active without rekindling old negative associations.

• Other physicians advocate swimming and walking. They argue that running and other strenuous activities, such as skiing, are too stressful for older joints.

Despite their differences, the experts agree on two basic points: Most of us need to be more active, and middle age is *not* too late to start.

"People are not lazy when it comes to activity," says Dr. Kuntzleman. "They simply have become accustomed to modern labor-saving devices. After a while, not moving becomes a force of habit." If you don't believe this, he recommends watching people in a parking lot or large airport. "People drive around for ten minutes looking for a space near the door. If they can't find one, some will even park in the space marked 'Handicapped Only' just to avoid walking a few extra feet. Similarly, when there's a choice between an escalator and stairs, ninety-nine out of a hundred people will take the easy way. I once actually saw people stand in line when an escalator temporarily stopped rather than take the stairs that were only two feet away."

Ironically, however, people tend to perceive themselves as being fairly active. They tend to equate their "hectic" life-styles with physical activity. They're active mentally, socially and in terms of their jobs, and they assume they are physically active as well.

To acquire a realistic grasp of how active you are, Dr. Kuntzleman suggests doing one or more of the following:

• Imagine going through an entire day without using any modern labor-saving devices. You will soon realize how inactive you are compared with your parents and your grandparents.

• For three days, keep close tabs on all of your activities. Write down exactly how much time you spend sleeping, sitting and moving about. Self-assessment like this usually proves that one overestimates activity and underestimates inactivity.

• Wear a pedometer for a few days, then compare how far you have actually walked with how far you think you have walked. A nurse who tried this test discovered that on the average she walked only one mile or slightly more than one mile on the job. She had estimated the distance at five or six miles.

The American College of Sports Medicine has issued four exercise guidelines for healthy adults. According to the College's official position statement, adhering to the guidelines will both train you for and maintain cardiovascular, pulmonary and musculoskeletal fitness. The recommendations for exercise are the following:

Frequency. Exercise a minimum of three and a maximum of five days per week.

Intensity. Exercise at a level that uses 60 to 90 percent of your maximum heart rate (this is roughly equivalent to 50 to 85 percent of your maximum oxygen intake, $V_{O_2}MAX$). To estimate your maximum heart rate, subtract your age from 220. If you are fifty years old, for example, your estimated maximum heart rate is 170 beats per minute. To determine your target zone pulse rate, multiply your estimated maximum heart rate by both .60 and .90. If you are fifty years old, the figure will be 170 multiplied by .60 and by .90 (102 and 153, respectively). Your target zone pulse rate at age fifty is between 102 and 153 beats per minute. If you are fifty-five years old, your maximum heart rate is 165 beats per minute, and your target pulse rate is between 99 and 148 beats per minute.

Duration. Do continuous, rhythmic activity for fifteen to sixty minutes. The less intense the activity, the longer it should be maintained.

Type of activity. Any activity should be engaged in that uses large muscle groups, is maintained continuously and is rhythmical in nature. These include running-jogging, walking-hiking, swimming, skating, bicycling and cross-country skiing. There are also weight-bearing and non-weight-bearing exercises. Weight-bearing exercises, such as jogging and skiing, are those that put additional stress on joints. Non-weight-bearing exercises, such as swimming, are recommended for those who are overweight, those just beginning an exercise program or those who have existing musculoskeletal or balance problems.

Isometric exercises are generally not recommended for older middle-aged adults, especially for those with a history of heart trouble or those who have high blood pressure. Isometrics are exercises that force muscles to contract but do not involve movement. They increase muscular strength but do not improve cardiovascular fitness. In some instances, they can even prove harmful. Isometric exercises tend to increase blood flow to specific muscle groups while diverting the blood supply away from vital body organs. If you have any doubt about whether or not to engage in isometric exercises, or in other specialized activities such as weight lifting and calisthenics, we suggest you check first with your physician.

How can you determine the amount of exercise necessary to meet your personal goals and expectations? According to Dr. Kuntzleman, a minimum workout of fifteen to thirty minutes, three times a week at the target heart rate will improve pulmonary and cardiovascular functions. To reduce body fat and to increase lean body tissue, you have to exercise at the target heart rate level for a minimum of thirty minutes, four times a week. To affect blood composition, you need to work out for forty to forty-five minutes, four times a week.

Before you change your exercise habits in any way, you should always consult with your physician first, whether or not you have a prior history of heart disease. According to Dr. Williams, some cardiovascular diseases, such as aortic stenosis (blockage of one of the heart valves) and high blood pressure, may be asymptomatic (without symptoms) in sedentary persons. But because they can be associated with a high risk of death or other adverse effects during exercise, it is important that you be screened for these problems.

You may need a routine physical examination, including an electrocardiogram and, possibly, a stress test (a treadmill or bicycle test that evaluates cardiovascular capacity during exertion). Your doctor can advise you on which tests you will need before you start an exercise program.

Once you decide to get started, which one of many exercises you choose to engage in is your personal choice. Your physician may suggest a specific regimen of activity: a timetable for walking, for example, or a specific number of laps in the pool. Exercise classes are also very good and help ensure compliance to an activity program. Before joining such a group:

• Sit in on one class and watch the participants. If they are primarily young go-getters, the class may be too quickly paced for you. Look for a group with a proportion of people your own age.
• Look for an instructor who is approximately your age.
• Ask the instructor to detail his or her objectives. If the answer is "to have a good time and improve cardiovascular fitness," this might be a good class for you.
• Ask class participants who are close to your age and fitness level how they feel about the program.
• Make sure the class has a warm-up period. In fact, you should schedule a ten- or fifteen-minute warm-up session before beginning any activity, except walking.

If you are in good health, you should be able to exercise relatively worry-free. No matter what your level of physical conditioning, however, it is important for you to know what danger signs to watch for. For example, excessive breathlessness is a sign of overexertion and means you should stop your activity immediately. Chest pain may be symptomatic of heart trouble. If it occurs, stop your activity and check with a physician before resuming any exercise. If you experience any discomfort in the upper neck or lower facial area, follow the same precautions as for chest pain.

Finally, keep tabs on how you feel after your activity is completed. If you are tired or short of breath the rest of the afternoon or evening, you are doing too much and need to cut back. If you feel very good one or two hours after your workout, then you are probably functioning at a level that is beneficial for you.

"Remember," says Dr. Kuntzleman, "exercise is not supposed to leave you exhausted. It is supposed to leave you revitalized."

HALL OF FAME FOR FIFTIES

Like Frank Sedgman in tennis, other masters continue to excel in their chosen sports. While famous athletes set sporting trends, many amateurs and lesser known men and women are following in the masters' footsteps. Here are just a few examples of the sporting world's "unsung heroes" of the fifties age group.

• Burton Morrow, D.D.S., a dentist from Cerritos, California, who, at age fifty-seven, beat his opponent 21–0 and 21–13 to retain his Golden Master's title at the National Racquetball Championships in Tempe, Arizona.

• Jim McElreath, of Arlington, Texas, who, at age fifty-two, became the oldest race-car driver to compete in the internationally famous Indianapolis 500.

• Ruth D. Christian, secretary and artist from Falls Church, Virginia, who, at age fifty-four, finished second in the division of women age fifty and over competing in the annual nationwide finals of the National Standard Race (NASTAR) slalom ski competition at Heavenly Valley, California. Christian, who won a silver medal for her efforts, did not begin skiing until she was forty-seven years old.

• Dean Westgaard, of Laguna Beach, California, a part-time Hollywood stuntman, who celebrated his fiftieth birthday by making the first legal parachute jump off the 3,600-foot-high El Captian rise in Yosemite National Park. Westgaard, a professor of physical education at Orange Coast College in California and an international parachute sales distributor, lists his hobbies as scuba diving, rock climbing, skydiving and white-water river running.

• James (Doc) Counselman, Ph.D., Indiana University swimming coach, who, at age fifty-eight, became the oldest person ever to swim the treacherous English Channel.

• Gail Peters Roper, former Olympic swimmer and now a fisheries technician from Los Altos, California, who, at age fifty, along with Jeannette Eppley, a former high school physical education teacher from Chicago, Illinois, age sixty, each won five events in the national Amateur Athletic Union (AAU) master's short-course swimming championships in Fort Lauderdale, Florida. Both women set new United States records for their respective age groups.

- William Minturn, M.D., a surgeon from Paradise Valley, Arizona, who, at age fifty-five, won both the Tucson and the Phoenix marathons in the fifty-five to fifty-nine age group. Minturn completed both races in one five-week period.

- Hank Rudolph, a sales promoter from Atlanta, Georgia, who, at age fifty-seven, shot two "Robin Hood split" arrows within forty-five minutes and at a distance of twenty yards, at a meet in College Park, Georgia. To shoot a Robin Hood split, the archer must hit the target with one arrow and then shoot a second arrow into the first, splitting it in half. Two weeks later, Rudolph won the Seniors' Southeastern Archery Championship in Greenville, South Carolina, and one month later, he captured the Georgia Seniors' Championship in Suwanee, Georgia. Rudolph had taken up archery only four and a half months before shooting the two Robin Hood splits. After shooting competitively for only 1½ years, Rudolph gave up shooting in just the seniors' ranks and tied for first overall in the Southeastern Archery Championship held in 1982 in Birmingham, Alabama.

- Dave Geer, a private contractor from Jewett City, Connecticut, who, at age fifty, captured the title of "World's Best Lumberjack" for the fourth time in competition held at Hayword, Wisconsin. Since winning his first championship in 1955, Geer has also won thirty-six national, state and local championships.

- John B. (Jack) Kelly, Jr., who, at age fifty-three, bested forty scullers to win first place in the Veteran's Singles competition for rowers age fifty and over, during the sixteenth showing of the Head of the Charles Regatta in Boston, Massachusetts. Kelly, also a triathlete, is a Philadelphia businessman and brother of the late Princess Grace (Kelly) Rainier of Monaco.

12

GUIDELINES FOR HEALTHY NUTRITION AND WEIGHT LOSS

"If physicians and nutritionists would agree on what they tell the public about diet, my life would be a lot simpler."

That was the comment made by a friend to Philip L. White, Sc.D., a nutrition expert with the American Medical Association. But who among us has not had similar thoughts?

The man who voiced that thought—Larry—was contemplating whether to end his birthday-party meal with baked Alaska or shaved chocolate cake. He had already enjoyed some wine, canapés and an Italian dinner. At age fifty, he is beginning to think about the process of aging, and of nutrition, which Dr. White discussed in an article in the *Journal of the American Medical Association.*

Although Larry is physically active and maintains appropriate weight for his height and build, he is aware of much of what has been written in the press about the relationship between diet and disease—and he is worried.

If you were in his situation, would you forego dessert? Listen to what Dr. White had to say:

His advice was to eat both, but in very small amounts. The serving of baked Alaska and shaved chocolate cake should be seen in relation to all other foods eaten that day and the next. After Larry had met his energy needs for the day, the desserts would be a surplus. But, since one has a single birthday each year, the slight excess would be unimportant.

Larry could burn up some of the excess calories exerting himself in celebratory dancing. Or he could cut down his calorie intake for the next few days to make up for the surplus, although that is not as much fun. However, when such modest excess becomes the rule, creeping obesity is the grim result, Dr. White said.

The point is that we each have decisions to make about what we eat and how much we eat. We do not all have nutrition experts to turn to for advice every time we face a tempting dessert. But out of the morass of confusing and often conflicting nutrition information—information that is rife with myth and fallacy—there are some sensible, prudent guidelines that are particularly germane to people in their fifties.

By this age, the rate at which cells in the human body use fuel supplied by food has slowed by a measurable amount. *Metabolism* is the term to describe the overall chemical processes that occur within cells. When these processes—actual chemical reactions—slow down, it is said that the metabolic rate declines. This happens normally with aging.

Metabolism and nutrition go hand in hand. You cannot have one without the other. The nutrients in food provide the energy, among other things, that allow the chemical process inside cells to take place. Nutrients from food also help form and maintain all the body tissues and they keep the internal environment supplied with essential substances so that the cells can function properly.

Even when we are at rest or asleep, our bodies require energy from the fuels in the diet or from fuels that have been stored when the diet supplies them in excess.

This energy is required to keep the body's temperature within normal limits, to keep the heart beating, to keep the muscles that inflate and deflate our lungs during breathing moving and to drive the chemical processes in the myriad cells that make up the human body.

By and large, we have little to do with our metabolism beyond supplying our bodies with the ingredients necessary for it to function. It would be an impossible task for each of us to look after our own metabolism, to control the thousands of chemical reactions that take place in our cells. Fortunately, we do not have to. Our nervous system, hormones and the special proteins called enzymes do it for us.

But there is one thing about our nutrition—besides supplying ourselves with nutrients—that we can look after. And that is our weight, which is an indication of how well we are balancing the fuel our bodies take in with the fuel they use up in metabolism.

Studies have revealed that there is a tendency among many of us to gain about one pound a year after age twenty-five. It doesn't take much to do this, only some ten extra calories a day above what we are required to consume to maintain our weight and energy expenditure. An extra doughnut a day—that's about 125 calories—will add thirteen pounds of fat in a year if your activity level is not increased to help compensate.

Calories have a mystique about them that is not entirely deserved. Most people know that certain foods have more calories than others, but beyond that, few of us know or remember what a calorie is or what it means to the body. Very simply, a calorie is a measurement of the energy value of food. When it is spelled with a capital C, as it is when nutritionists use it to compare foods, it stands for a kilocalorie. That is a term you need not bother remembering unless you are interested in the fact that it is the amount of heat required to raise the temperature of a kilogram of water by one degree centigrade.

The average adult requires some 500 calories during an eight-hour night of sleep and another 1,000 calories during the day just to provide energy for the right body temperature and all the other basic activities the body, its tissues and cells perform; in other words, for basal metabolism. Additional calories are required for additional activity or exercise.

We get these calories from the foods we eat or, more accurately, from the nutrients in these foods. The nutrients that supply calories are fats, carbohydrates and proteins.

The basic tenet of nutrition says that a sound diet provides our bodies with three things:

- The energy we need in the form of calories
- The building blocks to form and maintain body tissue
- The minerals and fluids we need to preserve the internal environment.

Proteins are not our chief source of calories. In the United States, it is estimated that approximately 15 percent of dietary calories are derived from protein. Besides calories, proteins supply our bodies with building blocks called amino acids, which are the constituents of food that help make and maintain body tissue. And, in that sense, proteins are more valuable to us for their building blocks than they are for their calories.

Our chief sources of calories are dietary fats and carbohydrates. In the typical American diet, about 40 percent of the calories are supplied by fats and 45 percent by carbohydrates. Just as we cannot do without protein for building blocks, we cannot do without carbohydrate or fat. These three nutrients are essential to our lives.

Add to these three the vitamins and minerals supplied by a balanced diet, and you have the five essentials of nutrition. They are essential simply because they must be supplied by the diet. From a handful of vitamins, minerals, amino acids, carbohydrates and fats—about forty-seven individual substances—the body can produce the thousands of substances involved in its metabolism. This is the marvel of our internal chemistry.

However, if we fail to provide an essential nutrient, be it a vitamin, a mineral or an amino acid, something will malfunction, causing a disorder known as a deficiency disease.

But what happens when we get too much of an essential nutrient? With the exception of a few vitamins, which can be stored in the body's fat tissue, and certain minerals, too much usually means too many calories. And too many calories can mean excess weight in the form of body fat, which is the way our bodies store energy reserves.

If protein provides the building blocks that are the structural basis for enzymes, for muscle and for the supporting matrix of tissue, then fats and carbohydrates provide the fuel on which our bodies run. Yet that is not all they do.

Carbohydrates from such dietary sources as cereals, flour or potatoes, and also fruits and vegetables, are the chief source of energy for the brain, which ounce for ounce requires proportionally more fuel than any other organ in the body. Other organs can utilize several different kinds of fuel, but the brain relies on a continuous and ample supply of carbohydrate.

Dietary fats serve in the formation of the sheathing that covers nerves, in the subcutaneous fat tissue that insulates our bodies and in the transportation and absorption of certain vitamins throughout the body. These vitamins are known as *fat-soluble*, and they include A, D, E and K. All the other vitamins are *water-soluble*.

No matter how they get in and around the body, however, all vitamins function essentially as helpers to speed or catalyze chemical reactions inside cells. Without an adequate supply of vitamins, certain vital chemical processes virtually grind to a halt, causing one or another vitamin-deficiency disease. Thus, fats serve several other functions besides contributing to our fuel supply by providing calories.

While we need both fats and carbohydrates, we do not need an overabundance of the calories they provide. And therein lies the rub. As most of us realize by looking in the mirror, it has not been all that difficult to gain excess weight. We have not purposely set out to add unneeded pounds, it has just happened that way. A nibble here, an extra helping there and slowly but surely the pounds add up. Not in one year or two or even five. But after ten or twenty years of virtually unconsciously eating a few extra calories a day, the weight is "suddenly" there.

What is often truly sudden, though, is our own recognition of the weight we have gained. It's not obvious, because when we look around at everybody else in our age group, everybody seems to have a bit of extra padding. That observation is not very far off the mark. In fact, studies show that the *most common* nutritional problem among adults in the United States is obesity. It has been estimated that more than half of us are overweight or obese.

If you are at the top end of the scale, you know where you stand. But even if you are not up there, you still may be overweight, and that extra ten or fifteen pounds of padding that have sneaked up on you, so to speak, are not doing you any good.

Compared with people of normal weight (see the "What You Should Weigh" chart on page 173), those who are overweight are more likely, researchers have found, to have high blood pressure, hardening of the arteries (known as arteriosclerosis), diabetes, gallbladder disease and hernia, to name a few conditions associated with the burden excess fat places on the body. On top of this, excess weight is known to aggravate heart disease and arthritis.

What you should weigh

Suggested Weights for Heights

Persons with wide shoulders and hips and large wrists and ankles can consider themselves in the "large frame" category. Those with narrow shoulders and hips and small wrists and ankles can consider themselves as having a "small frame." Most people fall in the "medium frame" category. Your estimated ideal weight should not change as you become older.

Feet & Inches	Small Frame	Medium Frame	Large Frame
	lbs	lbs	lbs
5'3"	118	129	141
5'4"	122	133	145
5'5"	126	137	149
5'6"	130	142	155
5'7"	134	147	161
5'8"	139	151	166
5'9"	143	155	170
5'10"	147	159	174
5'11"	150	163	178
6'	154	167	183
6'1"	158	171	188
6'2"	162	175	192
6'3"	165	178	195

Feet & Inches			
	lbs	lbs	lbs
5'	100	109	118
5'1"	104	112	121
5'2"	107	115	125
5'3"	110	118	128
5'4"	113	122	132
5'5"	116	125	135
5'6"	120	129	139
5'7"	123	132	142
5'8"	126	136	146
5'9"	130	140	151
5'10"	133	144	156
5'11"	137	148	161
6'	141	152	166

Source: *The Healthy Approach to Slimming*, © American Medical Association.

The specific disorders with which excess weight is associated had not been clearly identified in 1901 when Oscar H. Rogers of the New York Life Insurance Company began looking for risk factors that would help his company predict life span. In analyzing data from thousands of policyholders, he discovered that weight has a bearing on longevity. Policyholders of average weight, he found, lived longer than those who were overweight.

It was a simple yet startling association and it made ripples throughout the insurance business. It wasn't long after Rogers made his finding that Louis I. Dublin, who became the chief statistician at Metropolitan Life Insurance Company, started his personal crusade to get people to slim down. These efforts culminated when he coined the term *ideal weights* for a table he produced, which assigned people to one of three body builds or frame sizes. The concept of ideal weight gradually took hold.

In the intervening years, however, some segments of the population have taken the idea of slimming down to extremes. Mass-market advertising displays models who are, by the standards of the suggested height-weight tables, overly thin, encouraging a popular body image that is far different from the one Dublin probably had in mind.

In terms of creating a fashionable body image that many of us strive toward, the advertising has been remarkably successful, if misguided. There is, in the final analysis, no reason to be too thin. Striving for this body image creates its own hazards, not the least of which is the constant battle of mind over body.

Fad diets and quick-weight-loss regimens have boosted many authors to the best-seller lists, despite the fact that the diets are usually scientifically unsound and potentially dangerous. Low-protein diets can aggravate unsuspected kidney disease or heart problems. A diet severely deficient in fats can harm the efficiency at which glands function. Without fat, fat-soluble vitamins will not be transported or absorbed into the system, leading to a drying of the skin and scalp and a decrease in joint lubrication. High-fat diets can lead to diarrhea and associated loss of vitamins, minerals and other nutrients as the food passes through the body with too little opportunity to be fully absorbed.

The attention given to losing weight has a parallel in the pleasure we get from eating. If food, its preparation and its consumption were not as pleasurable as they are, we might not have to do as much battling with the bulge as we do. But eating is pleasurable, especially when we reach the stage of life in which we can sit back and enjoy our meals.

People who come up with diet schemes recognize this and they are aware of our desire to reconcile our appetite with the thin body image that looks out at us from billboards, television sets and magazines. Thus the proliferation of advice on dieting and losing weight.

If one diet really does work, you would expect that it would catch on. However, every year seems to bring a new solution. Unfortunately, no diet has ever improved on the basic tenet of weight reduction: You have to take in fewer calories than your system burns up.

Good food, by and large, is good for you; no diet should tell you otherwise. There is no reason for most people to alter their eating pattern radically as they get older. The only proviso—and the one that should apply at every stage of life—is to eat in moderation. This is one of the two keys to weight control.

The other is exercise, and the two go together.

The only other essential key is the key to sound nutrition. No one has yet come up with anything that approaches the soundness of eating foods from the four basic food groups: Milk, meat, bread-cereal and vegetable-fruit. Vitamin and mineral supplements, with few exceptions, are a waste of money. You'll get everything you need from a well-balanced diet, and if that sounds like an old saw, it is nevertheless a true old saw.

Proteins, for example, are combinations of some of the twenty known amino acids, eight of which are essential for adults because our bodies cannot form them. From different combinations of amino acids supplied by proteins in the diet, our cells re-form still other proteins that are used to produce enzymes and form and maintain body tissues. However, such protein can be formed only when all the constituent amino acids are present in the correct proportion. If one or more of the essential amino acids is missing —if it is not supplied by our diet, that is—the body cannot make all the protein it needs.

Some proteins have a more complete amino acid combination than others, at least in terms of what is required by our bodies.

When nutritionists speak of high-grade protein or a complete protein, they are referring to those proteins—specifically from meat, fish or eggs—that have amino acid combinations similar to those needed by the human body.

Vegetable protein—from beans or peas, for instance—is of somewhat lower quality, only because its combination of amino acids is not as closely matched to our requirements as is the combination found in animal protein sources.

Nevertheless, two or more proteins, each lacking a different essential amino acid, can complement one another when consumed together. That is one reason why the American Medical Association advocates eating a variety of foods. It is the best way to a sound diet, one that provides the essentials of good nutrition.

You might have heard or read that keenness of taste declines with age and wondered whether or not this is a subtle message that the body sends out to tell us that food is not as important to the system as it used to be when we were younger.

First of all, our requirements for the essential nutrients do not appreciably decrease with age. We need to eat right during every stage of life.

The only adjustment we need to make as we get older is to reduce our intake of calories (or increase our energy expenditure) to compensate for our reduced energy needs. Just walk by a school yard at recess and you'll get some impression of why the energy needs of youngsters are higher than yours.

Second, the widely held belief that our sensitivity to taste wanes with age is turning out to be a myth. The latest research, conducted under the auspices of the National Institute on Aging, shows that our taste perception remains remarkably consistent no matter how old we are.

In essence, our bodies are not sending us any messages about the need for food, other than those that tell us when we are hungry, when we are sated and when things taste good.

Losing Weight and Satisfying Nutritional Needs

The experts who specialize in aging say that people in their fifties face two dietary challenges: They have to assess whether or not they need to cut calories, and they need to maintain an adequate level of the essential nutrients.

The importance of cutting calories if you need to is a subject that has been addressed in laboratory studies on animals. In research again sponsored by the National Institute on Aging, investigators have found that animals on a diet restricted only in the total number of calories consumed daily lived longer than animals given unlimited access to food. What's more, the animals on a restricted-calorie diet developed fewer tumors than did the animals that were freely fed.

While no one is saying that these findings can be directly translated to human experience, they do give one pause to think—and, of course, they are stimulating further studies into the question of diet and aging. Nevertheless, research that has been substantiated in humans shows that our basal metabolic rate (the rate at which the cells of our body use the fuel supplied by food) declines with age. So does our energy expenditure in physical activity.

Simply said, the cells of our body slow down, and so do we as we age. Nothing about it is tragic; it is as normal a physiological process as the adjustments our bodies went through during adolescence.

Unfortunately some habits die hard, and though we might not need as many calories as we did when we were younger, the amount of high-caloric food we eat usually does not reflect the adjustments our bodies are making. The consequences of this imbalance can be measured in belt notches.

An important point to realize is that we don't have to overeat to gain weight, not at least to gain it slowly. All we have to do is eat like we always used to, and by the time we reach age fifty we have long exceeded our ideal weight. It seems that our bodies are more finely attuned to adjust for taking in more calories than they are in making an adjustment to fewer calories.

Because it can creep up on us so slowly, such weight gain seems reasonable if it has not gotten out of hand. But medical evidence has shown that extra pounds put additional strain on every organ of the body. The more fat cells we have in the body, the more blood we are diverting from vital organs. This puts a load on the heart muscle, forcing it to work harder to supply the body's needs while also depriving other organs of needed fuel.

Ask yourself whether or not your eating habits have changed in the last ten, twenty or thirty years? Add up how often and how long you exercise. And then take a good, long look at yourself in the mirror. If you are like most people in their fifties, you'll notice that the amount of fat tissue has increased over what it was when you were younger. Beneath the fat, there has also been a loss of muscle or lean body tissue.

The normal decline in the metabolic rate—estimated at about 15 percent between the ages of thirty and eighty—is responsible for these shifts in body composition. Even if you've watched your weight and exercised, these changes take place. The only difference is in degree.

Adjusting your calorie intake to meet your body's reduced metabolic rate is part of the formula for achieving the proper weight in your fifties and thereafter. But there is also another reason why you may need to cut back on calories. The actual number of calories you use up in physical activity tends to dwindle with age. One study on this phenomenon showed that the average male expended 1,166 calories a day when he was between the ages of thirty-five and forty-four. But, by the time he was in his fifties, this figure had dropped to about 950.

Of course, your own calorie expenditure is dependent upon your own level of activity, so, if you're very active or exercise regularly, don't go by the figures cited for the average male. You'll have to find out what is right for you.

We can offer some guidance, however. The National Academy of Sciences/National Research Council suggests a 10 percent reduction in calories after age fifty for those of you whose physical activity is light or if you are generally sedentary.

If you are moderately active, the World Health Organization advocates a 5 percent reduction in calories for each decade between the ages of forty and fifty-nine, and a 10 percent decrease between sixty and sixty-nine years of age.

The mathematics of weight reduction is based on a simple time-honored formula that most of the popular diet books seem to overlook. On one side of the equation is the number of calories in minus the number of calories out. On the other side of the equal sign is a plus or minus figure or zero.

If you want to lose weight, you either have to consume fewer calories or exercise more or, preferably, do both. There is no other way, despite what the diet books lead you to believe. And no shortcuts really work.

Diets that boast quick weight loss usually achieve nothing initially but water loss. True, water weighs something, but you'll put the pounds right back on. And having your weight go up and down hardly provides a sound foundation from which to learn a better way of eating.

To be realistic in losing more than, say, ten pounds, you should think in terms of months or even a year instead of weeks. If you're aiming at a faster weight loss—and even if you're not—you ought to consult with your family physician and have a physical examination before embarking on any diet, even one in which you are only reducing the number of calories.

It's a good idea to keep your new diet as normal as possible, while getting the benefits of a lower caloric intake from low-fat and nonfat dairy products, leaner cuts of meat, smaller servings of snacks and desserts and anything else that has a high calorie value (such as alcoholic beverages).

If you have trouble conceptualizing what calories actually are, think of them as the basic quantity of fuel necessary to keep you alive, alert and functioning in your daily activities. Most people leading moderately active lives need about fifteen calories—or units of fuel—per pound of body weight to maintain their weight. For instance, a 150-pound individual needs no more than 2,250 calories a day to maintain proper weight. More calories than that, with no offsetting exercise, means weight gain, as the excess fuel is converted into deposits of fat.

Each pound of fat contains some 3,500 calories. So you can figure that, if you want to lose ten pounds, you need to expend 35,000 calories more than you consume. If you expect to lose this much weight in a month, let's say, you'll need to reduce your calorie intake and increase your exercise so as to have a daily deficit of between 1,300 and 1,400 calories.

This can mean a considerable change in your life-style if you are planning to lose this much weight over such a short time. But if you plan to lose only one pound a month, you won't have to make such major adjustments. Just skip one slice of bread a day from what you had been eating. Or forego a tablespoonful of margarine.

A sensible weight-loss program, conducted over many months, can help break old patterns of eating, and break them for good—

something the fad diets have never achieved. All in all, slow and steady is the best course when it comes to dieting, and this is especially true for people in their fifties, a time when crash dieting can be potentially harmful.

One definitely wrong approach to cutting calories is to skip meals. This puts stress on the body to function without readily available supplies of its needed fuel, in the form of blood sugar (glucose). Besides, it doesn't work very well anyway, because you will then tend to overindulge at the next meal.

The trick to cutting calories in your fifties, while maintaining a proper nutrient level, is to watch those foods high in fats and carbohydrates. But that does not mean that you have to cut them out entirely.

You might have heard, among other myths about dieting, that some foods help you lose weight because they are burned up faster than others. That's nutritional nonsense, even though it helps sell diet books. There is no law against preaching unsound information about diet. But if you judge all such claims against the fact that the only way to lose weight is to take in fewer calories than you use, you'll find your way to firm nutritional ground.

Few myths and fallacies about nutrition can stand up to the one simple fact that it is total calories—and not the foods they come from—that make the difference between gaining and losing weight.

Even so, it is well to bear in mind that fats are the most concentrated source of calories. One gram of fat contains nine calories versus four calories per gram of protein. Sugars and starches, which biochemists and nutritionists call carbohydrates, are no more concentrated a source of calories than protein.

To put this in perspective, let's go back to that tablespoonful of margarine. It contains about 11.3 grams of fat, which translates to 100 calories. Gram for gram, this is more than twice as much as in carbohydrate and protein, so you can see why, if you're cutting calories, it pays to keep a close eye on serving sizes of foods high in fat.

A daily diet selected from among foods in the four basic groups —milk, meat, bread-cereal and vegetable-fruit—will provide you with all the essentials necessary for good nutrition. If some extra fat creeps into your diet through the use of butter, margarine or oils, it won't spoil what you've set out to accomplish unless you are immoderate in the use of such items.

Meat, fish, poultry and eggs will supply protein, fat and certain B-group vitamins. Peas, beans and nuts also supply protein. Whole milk and whole-milk products, such as cheese, supply calcium and riboflavin (a vitamin) as well as protein and fat. Green and yellow vegetables supply vitamin A and minerals. Along with cereals, potatoes, flour and rice, they also supply carbohydrate, the major brain fuel. Tomatoes and citrus fruits supply vitamin C. For a more complete listing of nutrients and where to find them, consult the chart on page 182.

Contrary to another nutritional belief, people in their fifties do not require more protein than they did when they were younger. So, if you're one of those people who tends to eat twice as much meat as you need to get your protein, remember that two to three *ounces* of meat equals one serving.

Diet—and that means the foods you eat—is not the whole answer to physical well-being. Certainly, exercise and adequate rest play important roles. But if you have to start somewhere—and let's face it, who doesn't?—eat a little less of everything that you do eat. That's not very much in the way of a sacrifice to ask of yourself when you consider that the potential benefits are a healthier, longer life.

Losing Weight—A New Body Image

"Why do you want to lose weight?"

Every patient who walks through the doors of the health and weight clinic at Johns Hopkins Hospital, Baltimore, Maryland, is asked that question. In the past several years, more than 20,000 people—ranging from adolescents to senior citizens—have answered, and their responses have been overwhelmingly the same: "I want to look better."

"We've developed a slim cult," says Maria Simonson, Sc.D., who heads the program and who has worked with more than 43,000 men and women who wanted to lose weight. "Our society today has put a premium on looking like Madison Avenue models, and that's unfortunate." Only recently, she notes, has there been an indication of a change in thinking. Now the individuals who

Nutrients: Where To Find Them

Nutrient	Important Sources of Nutrient	What they do for you
Protein	Meat, poultry, fish, dried beans and peas, eggs, milk, cheese	Constitutes part of the structure of every cell such as muscle, blood, and bone; supports growth and maintains healthy body cells.
Vitamin A	Liver, carrots, sweet potatoes, greens, butter, margarine	Assists formation and maintenance of skin and mucous membranes that line the body cavities and tracts, such as nasal passages and intestinal tract, thus increasing resistance to infection.
Vitamin C	Broccoli, oranges, papaya, grapefruit, mango, strawberries	Forms cementing substances, such as collagen, that hold body cells together, thus strengthening blood vessels, hastening healing of wounds and bones and increasing resistance to infection.
Thiamin (B_1)	Lean pork, nuts, fortified cereal products	Aids in utilization of energy. Contributes to normal functioning of nervous system.
Riboflavin (B_2)	Liver, milk, yogurt, cottage cheese	Aids in utilization of energy. Promotes healthy skin and eyes.
Niacin	Liver, peanuts, meat, fish, poultry, fortified cereal products	Aids in utilization of energy. Aids digestion and fosters normal appetite.
Calcium	Milk, yogurt, cheese, sardines and salmon with bones, collard, kale, turnip and mustard greens	Combines with other minerals within a protein framework to give structure and strength to bones and teeth.
Iron	Enriched farina, red meat, prune juice, liver, dried beans and peas	Combines with protein to form hemoglobin, the red substance in blood that carries oxygen to and carbon dioxide from the cells. Prevents nutritional anemia and its accompanying fatigue. Increases resistance to infection.
Vitamin D	Vitamin D milk, fish, liver, oils, sunshine on skin (not a food)	Helps absorb calcium from the digestive tract and builds calcium and phosphorus into bone.
Vitamin E	Vegetable oils, green leafy vegetables, whole grain cereals, wheat germ, butter, egg yolk, milkfat	Protects vitamin A and unsaturated fatty acids from destruction by oxygen. Exact biochemical mechanism by which it functions still unknown.
Vitamin B_6	Beef, liver, pork, ham, lima beans, bananas, whole grain cereals	Assists in red blood cell regeneration. Helps regulate the use of protein, fat, and carbohydrate.

Nutrient	Important Sources of Nutrient	What they do for you
Folic Acid (Folacin)	Green leafy vegetables, liver, dry legumes, nuts, whole grain cereals, some fruits such as oranges	Assists in normal blood formation. Helps enzyme and other biochemical systems function.
Vitamin B$_{12}$	Only in animal foods—liver, meat, fish, shellfish, milk, milk products, eggs, poultry. Vegetarian diets should include milk or a B$_{12}$ supplement	Assists in the maintenance of nerve tissues and normal blood formation.
Phosphorus	Milk and milk products, meat, poultry fish, eggs, whole grain cereals, legumes	Combines with calcium to give bones and teeth strength. Helps regulate many internal activities of the body.
Iodine	Seafoods, iodized salt	Helps regulate the rate at which the body uses energy.
Magnesium	Legumes, whole grain cereals, milk, meat, nuts, seafood, eggs, green vegetables	Helps regulate the use of carbohydrate and production of energy within the cells. Helps nerves and muscles work.
Zinc	Meat, liver, eggs, oysters, other seafoods, milk, whole grain cereals	Becomes part of several enzymes and insulin.

Reproduced from "Recommended Dietary Allowances," (9th Edition) 1980, with permission of the National Academy of Sciences, Washington, D.C.

went first to commercial groups and fast-weight-loss promoters to improve appearance are coming to the Hopkins clinic for the sake of improving their health.

"Today approximately 60 percent of the people who come to the Baltimore clinic do so for health reasons. In the past, health considerations ranked far down the list as reasons for wanting to lose weight." Dr. Simonson considers the change a major step in the right direction. "We are finally more conscious of health," she explains. "We may also be beginning to realize that we needn't be a nation of slim models or Twiggies."

We have already discussed the link between good health and proper weight, an issue that becomes especially important for people in their fifties. It is at this point that many weight problems develop.

"If you were to draw a graph tracing activity levels and weight gains from age twenty to about age sixty, you would see the activity level very high at twenty, then dropping sharply. Weight is relatively low at age twenty and climbs slowly for many years. Eventually the two lines meet and cross—usually around fifty years of age. That's when activity falls way down and weight goes up sharply. It's an 'X-rated' time, and you should be aware of it," says Dr. Simonson.

A bit of honest self-appraisal can help you to lose weight. Ask a friend or family member to snap several candid shots at the next group get-together and then look at yourself and run a critique. One middle-aged man never believed he was overweight until he saw a photo of himself taken at a wedding. The picture could not hide the fifty extra pounds he was carrying on his frame. Better still, though maybe more difficult, is to face yourself in the flesh before a full-length mirror. Decide, realistically, with this evidence staring back at you, whether you feel you are a healthy, physically fit person for your age.

But even this technique demands caution. One 305-pound man found he could continue to rationalize his weight as long as he faced the mirror head-on. In his own eyes, he looked only large and heavyset, until he turned sideways and viewed himself from another angle. Disturbed by his "balloon" profile, he finally began to diet.

If you wonder whether you are overweight, ask yourself the following questions:

- Do I feel good?
- Do I have vague aches and pains?
- Am I slowing down?
- Do I tend to eat when I am tense?

If you answer no to the first question and yes to the last three, you might have a weight problem.

The first thing you should do is go to your family physician for a complete checkup. If you need to lose weight, start and follow a weight-reduction program established and supervised by your doctor. This advice is appropriate for people who want to lose ten pounds as well as for those who want to lose 100, says Dr. Simonson. "Maybe I'm overly strict, but in eleven years I have seen some bad results from people who have gone overboard on their own."

At the Center for Nutritional Research, Boston, Massachusetts; at the Dietary Rehabilitation Clinic, Durham, North Carolina; at the Johns Hopkins Clinic, Baltimore, Maryland; and at many of the hospital-affiliated obesity and weight-reduction centers in the country, emphasis falls on two principles: sound nutrition and regular exercise. The link between the two is indisputable.

Marion Hendricks, a fifty-three-year-old California realtor, lost eight pounds and a total of fifteen inches from her figure. "I found myself looking matronly and didn't like it, so I decided to do something about it," says Marion. She'd been on diet binges in the past and, in spurts, had gotten involved in basic exercise programs. This time she combined the two forces and achieved her goal.

"Anyone can do what I did if they want to," says Marion, the mother of four grown children. Marion went to a weight-loss counselor for help and direction because she recognized the need to break out of old patterns of cooking, eating and inactivity, not only to lose weight but to keep the weight off. In effect, she set up a pattern (new eating habits, a varied activity schedule) for a potentially new model of herself. By following the pattern, she made the model a reality.

We can all alter our behavior and our body image as Marion Hendricks did if we understand how the process of behavior change works, says Louis Jolyon West, M.D., director of the neuropsychiatric institute at the University of California, Los Angeles. "You have to decide what the behavior is you want to change. Then you measure it until certain patterns emerge. When you understand the pattern, you can take the steps to break it."

Measuring behavior means keeping a log or diary. Write down every instance of undesirable behavior, such as snacking or skipping meals. Note the date, time and reinforcing or accompanying circumstances. Do this for at least two weeks, preferably for four, and you will discover your own particular pattern of behavior.

A typical example might be the following: An overweight man has faithfully followed a daily dietary routine of going without breakfast, drinking coffee all morning and eating no lunch (he's "too busy" and works through the noon hour). Once home, he immediately fixes a drink in the family room, then walks to the kitchen and eats 2,000 calories in snacks before dinner.

To break the pattern, the man can do something as simple as changing his clothes as soon as he comes home from work, then going for a walk around the block. Thus he postpones—and maybe eliminates—the drink, gets some exercise and most importantly sets up a pattern of behavior for a different self. This approach, which is now well documented in publications on behavior therapy, can be used both for behavior you want to decrease —such as drinking or eating—and for behavior you want to increase—such as exercise.

Losing weight can be more difficult during middle age than during earlier stages of life, but it is not an impossible goal. In order to maintain or to re-establish a proper, healthful weight at middle age, you need to understand the factors that are working against you. You need to recognize that a slowed metabolic rate, decreased physical activity and a social environment that promotes the often excessive consumption of food and calorie-rich alcohol are primarily responsible for the problem of "creeping pounds" that may plague you. You also need to realize that these elements are factors you can control, as discussed in this chapter and in Chapter 2.

Unfortunately, many middle-aged adults suffer from the misconception that they are overweight because they are "compulsive eaters," says Albert J. Stunkard, M.D., professor of psychiatry at the University of Pennsylvania, Philadelphia, and the author of *The Pain of Obesity* (Bull Publishing Company, 1980). The label allows overweight individuals to resign themselves to being overweight, and it also provides a convenient excuse for their often unhealthy eating habits.

Thus the man who loads up a platter of goodies from a food-laden brunch table says he does so because he cannot help himself. The woman who inevitably consumes both doughnuts and pastries at coffee break says she "just has to have a bite of something sweet."

"People who follow this pattern of behavior may think they are victims of an eating compulsion, but they are not," says Dr. Stunkard. "In fact, their actions are very different from those of the true compulsive or binge eater."

A true compulsive eater is one who, although aware that such behavior is not normal, participates in episodic eating binges and goes to great lengths to procure food if none is readily available. The compulsive eater eats furtively and rapidly, gobbling easily consumable, often sweet and gooey foods. The compulsive eater also fears not being able to stop eating voluntarily. Usually he eats until overcome by sleep or intense abdominal pain. He may even induce vomiting to relieve his discomfort or to relieve the guilt he feels at having consumed thousands of unnecessary calories. When the binge is over, the compulsive eater is depressed and suffers from self-deprecating thoughts. He often feels his entire life is dominated by conflicts related to food and eating.

Among the obese, compulsive eaters represent only about 5 percent of the total population. Among people with eating disorders, compulsive eating is much more common in younger people than it is in the middle-aged. When it occurs, the problem is often difficult to manage and requires extensive medical supervision.

For the most part, people in the fifties age group who are ten or twenty pounds overweight are *not* compulsive eaters. For them, the term is not only inappropriate but also detrimental, because it connotes an overriding sense of powerlessness and helplessness.

The real problem for most overweight middle-aged individuals is that they react to temptation. They eat more food than they need to because the food is there; they consume more alcohol than they should because the alcohol is there. Once you become aware of how your environment affects your eating and drinking habits, you can begin to understand how to cope with the situation. Then you will discover that your weight problems, like those of most middle-aged people, are quite manageable.

How can you lose weight successfully? According to Dr. Simonson, you need three ingredients, what she calls a weight-loss trilogy. The base of the trilogy is made up of sound nutrition. Combined with this is a sensible, ongoing program of physical activity. The third factor in the trilogy is self-awareness. Self-awareness comes from introspection, from keeping a careful log of behavior (a prerequisite for patients at the Johns Hopkins weight-loss clinic) and, for some individuals, from professional counseling. "Really being aware of yourself—your motives, your actions, the benefits you'll achieve by losing weight—is vital," says Dr. Simonson. "It's a complex process. Basic to it is that you have to know yourself and accept the responsibility for taking care of yourself and your health."

13

MAKING A
DECISION ABOUT
COSMETIC SURGERY

*I don't think I need cosmetic surgery yet, but if suddenly
everything started drooping, I'd get a face-lift. My friends
wouldn't approve. It's that Depression-era outlook that says
spending money on your face is frivolous, and I might have
some problems with that, too. But I'd do it anyway. The way
I feel about myself is important, and if a face-lift would
make me feel better, then fine.*

—a fifty-year-old high school teacher

For increasing numbers of middle-aged men and women, looking
better and feeling better about themselves means undergoing some
form of cosmetic or aesthetic surgery. Every year an estimated
400,000 people—many of them in their fifties—submit to what
was once called vanity surgery, but now is being increasingly
accepted as a valid, elective procedure.

"It's permissible now for people to care about their appearance,
and society has given them greater freedom in what is accepted,"
explains John M. Goin, M.D., clinical professor of surgery at the
University of Southern California School of Medicine, Los Angeles. "Ten years ago, patients asked if I had a back door they
could use so that they wouldn't be seen coming here. Now many
go to work and show off their stitches."

There's a growing tendency to feel that having your face lifted
or eyelids tucked is a perfectly normal thing to do. There's also
a trend away from thinking that cosmetic surgery is only for the

wealthy or the famous. Among a group of recent face-lift patients that Dr. J. Goin treated were several secretaries, teachers and hairstylists, as well as a woman barber and a letter carrier.

The most common procedures among middle-aged patients are the rhytidectomy (face-lift), the blepharoplasty (eyelid tuck) and reduction mammoplasty (breast reduction). (See the charts starting on page 192 for a description of the more common forms of plastic surgery, along with age-related guidelines.) With the exception of the breast reduction, none of these operations alters the basic composition of the individual's appearance, but all help to erase or ease some of the wrinkles, tensions and sags of time. Although they will not make you look different, they will make you look better, and this is an important consideration.

"Do I look tired?" a prospective face-lift patient asks the physician. "Do I seem dissipated and worn out?" Men considering the eyelid tuck often explain that "my eyes are so baggy, people always ask if I had a rough night or really hung one on the evening before." Women seeking breast reduction complain of back and shoulder pain, difficulty buying clothes and limited activity.

Not too surprisingly, concerns about career and work-related issues often prompt the middle-aged to seek cosmetic surgery. When asked why she wanted a face-lift, one woman explained, "If something happened to my husband that placed me in financial jeopardy, I would feel more confident in my ability to find employment."

Another patient had worked as a secretary for many years for the same boss. When he retired and was replaced by a younger man, she became convinced the new boss would want a more youthful assistant. The woman decided on a face-lift and after the operation told her surgeon that now her boss thought she was great. "He listens to everything I say," she explained with great enthusiasm. But, as the surgeon pointed out, the face-lift didn't change the boss; it only changed the patient's perception of herself.

"The work issue is very subtle," says Dr. J. Goin. "Patients—and often they are men—think that the boss is about to fire them or that someone else will be promoted over them simply because the other person looks younger. Now, this may not be true at all, but the person feels that way and reacts to it. Such people may become sullen. Their work deteriorates. A face-lift helps them to feel better, so they function better, and often their work situation improves." In many instances middle-aged men and women seek aesthetic surgery to alter situations that have bothered them for years. If they can afford the time and money for elective surgery, they do so.

Just recently, for example, Dr. J. Goin performed surgery on a fifty-five-year-old woman, a self-employed accountant, who wanted silicone breast implants to enlarge what she'd always considered a too-small bosom. The woman was delighted, says the surgeon, with the results of what he considers an unusual procedure for a woman her age.

For women who have undergone a mastectomy, another procedure, called breast reconstruction, can provide a positive, supportive means for dealing with the trauma of breast cancer. Dr. J. Goin and Marcia Kraft Goin, M.D., professor of psychiatry and the behavorial sciences at the University of Southern California School of Medicine, Los Angeles, recently completed a joint study of seventeen mastectomy/breast-reconstruction patients, 70 percent of whom had completed the menopause. They found repeated examples of women who had pretended, some for years, that losing a breast to a mastectomy had not bothered them. Outwardly they had coped well and were back at work or active again in the community. But inwardly they had first been depressed by their loss and then ashamed because of their reaction. "These things are not supposed to matter to a woman of my age," said one woman. Another woman who had a breast reconstruction operation told Dr. M. Goin, "Now I don't have to fear that my husband is staying with me out of pity."

Motivations for cosmetic surgery are often complex and are sometimes not even realized on a conscious level until after surgery. That is when the woman who had the face-lift, ostensibly to improve her chin line, admits that she had secretly hoped her operation would cure her husband's indifference. Or the man who says he wanted to eliminate baggy eyelids owns up to the fact that he really hoped to develop a new, more outgoing personality because of the operation. Most plastic surgeons agree that the best motivation is knowingly and willingly to seek the surgery for yourself, and not to save a faltering marriage, impress a boss or get

Cosmetic Surgery: How It's Done

E very year in the United States, an estimated 400,000 men and women, many of them in their fifties, undergo some kind of aesthetic, or cosmetic, surgery. The most common procedures among middle-aged adults are the rhytidectomy (face lift), blepharoplasty (the eyelid tuck) and reduction mammaplasty (breast reduction).

On the following pages you will find explanations of these and other common cosmetic surgery procedures.

NAME	PURPOSE	HOW IT'S DONE	GUIDELINES
Chemosurgery (Face peeling)	Eliminates fine wrinkles, surface scars and pigmented spots.	Chemical formula, painted on skin, reacts with upper layers of skin to produce superficial chemical burn. Treated skin area peels away.	For all adult age groups.
Augmentation mammaplasty (Breast surgery)	Enlarges breasts.	Incision is made under breast, around nipple, or in armpit area. Silicone prosthesis (an artificial device) is placed behind breast to enlarge it and push it forward.	Most common among women ages 20-40.
Reduction mammaplasty (Breast surgery)	Reduces breast size.	Portion of breast tissue is removed. Breast is reshaped and nipple repositioned.	For all adult age groups. Most common among women ages 25-50.
Reconstruction mammaplasty (Breast surgery)	Rebuilds breasts (see illustrations, below).	Incision is made in skin (fig. 1); silicone prosthesis or saline-filled sac is implanted to form the new breast (fig. 2). Physician sews incision and fashions new nipple.	For traumatic breast deformities or for mastectomy patients. For all adult age groups.

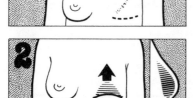

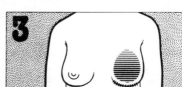

Breast remaking (reconstruction mammaplasty) is performed to correct traumatic breast deformities or to reconstruct the breast after a mastectomy.

NOTE: Material was developed in cooperation with Donald R. Klein, M.D., of the Plastic Surgery Center of Dallas, Texas. It is intended for general informational purposes only.

Anyone who is considering cosmetic surgery procedures and has questions should consult his or her personal physician.

NAME	PURPOSE	HOW IT'S DONE	GUIDELINES
Rhytidectomy (Face lift)	Tightens sagging skin around cheeks, chin and neck. Helps eliminate wrinkles (see illustrations, below).	Incision is made at the temple, around the front of the ear and back toward the neck (fig. 2, below). Supportive structures of face and neck, including muscle layer, are manipulated and sometimes cut and stitched for a better framework on which to stretch the skin (fig. 3). Skin is trimmed and sewn along incision line (fig. 4).	Usually for adults age 30 on up.

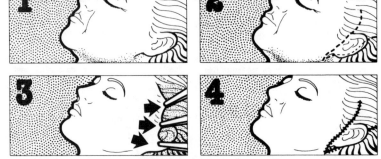

The face lift (rhytidectomy) tightens sagging skin and helps eliminate wrinkles.*

NAME	PURPOSE	HOW IT'S DONE	GUIDELINES
Rhinoplasty (Nose reconstruction)	Eliminates bump in nose, and can straighten, shorten or lengthen nose.	Cartilage of nose is cut and reshaped. Skin is stretched and cut to conform to new shape.	Can be done at any age.
Otoplasty (Ear reshaping)	Prominent ears are repositioned.	Incision is made behind ear. Cartilage of ear is reshaped and incision is sewn.	Generally performed on children and young adults, but not limited to those age groups.

*NOTE: Dashed lines indicate incision lines. Crossed lines are suture or stitched areas.

NAME	PURPOSE	HOW IT'S DONE	GUIDELINES
Blepharoplasty (Eyelid tuck)	Tightens drooping eyelids and eliminates bags under eyes (see illustrations below).	Incision is made above the lash line (fig. 2). Excess skin and fat are removed. Skin is sewn (fig. 3). Procedure is then repeated on lower lid (figs. 4 and 5).	Most common for ages 45-60. (May be indicated for earlier age groups.)

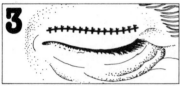
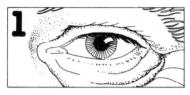
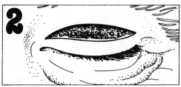
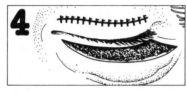
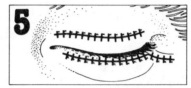
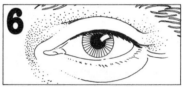

The eyelid tuck (blepharoplasty) is a common cosmetic surgery procedure for both men and women in middle age.

NAME	PURPOSE	HOW IT'S DONE	GUIDELINES
Body Sculpting (Surgery on upper arms, midriff, thighs, abdomen or buttocks.)	Removes excess skin and fat.	Procedure varies. Patient must be willing to accept scarring, which will fade with time. Results for the patient can be dramatic.	For some formerly very obese individuals or for those who have lost skin elasticity.
Hair transplant	Eliminates some baldness.	Hair is grafted from one portion of scalp to the balding area.	Generally not indicated for individuals over age 50.

a new job. This can sometimes present a tricky problem in the surgeon's consulting room, where the wife sits, eager for a face-lift, and the husband intones in a self-righteous manner that "she looks fine; she doesn't have to do this for me." The issue becomes even more sensitive when breast reconstruction is discussed.

It is possible for a spouse to react in a variety of ways to this kind of operation. He may feel he has somehow failed and not been supportive enough of his wife through the initial surgery for breast cancer. He may argue that his wife has already undergone the trauma of surgery (the mastectomy) and he does not want her to go through another operation for his sake. He may fear unsatisfactory results from the surgery, sure that his wife will then be bitter toward him—the "I did it for you" syndrome.

"It comes as a revelation to the husband that the woman is doing this for herself—even if *he* doesn't mind, *he* likes her anyway. He realizes then that this is important to *her*. It has nothing to do with him at all. It's not his fault that she feels bad and wants her breast back. He becomes aware of how much this means to her," says Dr. M. Goin.

Because eyelid tucks and face-lifts counter natural aging processes, they are, of course, associated with a desire for a more youthful, firmer appearance. Even here there are fine lines to be crossed. Wanting to *look* younger is not the same as wanting to *be* younger. The first is a legitimate expectation of cosmetic surgery. The other is not. "If people think a face-lift is going to make them younger, that they'll be more vital and more vigorous, then they are bound to be disappointed," says Dr. J. Goin.

Cosmetic surgery is not a panacea, a magic door to another world, though some people try to use it that way, like the Indiana computer programmer who, at age forty-nine, according to local legend, got a divorce, a face-lift, an eyelid tuck, a rhinoplasty, new cheekbones and a dimpled chin. He quit his job, gave away his business suits, sold his house and left for the South Seas—sporting a silver necklace and a silky shirt opened halfway down his chest.

"That's coping with a mid-life crisis by creating a new self, and it doesn't work," says Dr. M. Goin. "It's attempting to deny that one is growing older. It's saying, 'I won't accept that, I will be a whole new person instead.' But you are who you are, and you do continue to age. You have to come to terms emotionally with the problems of mid-life and with the issue of personal mortality. The other way out is just running away, and one thing you can't run away from is getting old."

What you can do, however, is say to yourself, "This operation is going to make me look younger, and I'll feel better if I look younger. It's going to cause me to look refreshed, and if I look more refreshed, I will feel better about myself." As for those who argue that aging should not be denied and that a face-lift is, in fact, attempting to deny the natural process of life, then the feelings of such people should be respected. "No one should have to be talked into cosmetic surgery," says Dr. M. Goin.

Is it a question of vanity to want aesthetic surgery? You will hear some people argue that it is: Norman E. Hugo, M.D., of Northwestern University Medical School, Chicago, Illinois, tells patients, no, it is not. "I explain that vanity is wanting to look like someone else, a movie star, maybe, but that to want to look like yourself is not vanity. Aesthetic surgery won't make you pretty or handsome if you are not. Most likely it will make you look like you did several years ago."

Aesthetic surgery, then, is an attempt to bring reality into line with your image of yourself. For the most part, society today accepts and even encourages this trend.

But before you commit yourself to cosmetic surgery, there are certain things you should know. For the most part, age itself is not a criterion for determining whether or not you should have aesthetic surgery, but health is a major consideration. The basic guideline is simple: You should be in reasonably good health to undergo elective surgery of any kind. Doctors list four conditions that might preclude aesthetic surgery for the middle-aged. Malignant disease is one. So, too, is severe heart disease, when the risk of doing harm to the person outweighs the possible benefits. Severe hypertension, in the range of 150–160 over 100–110, can cause excessive bleeding, a potentially disasterous complication. (Once the blood pressure is brought under control, however, surgery can be done quite safely.) Also important are the types of medications you may be taking, and this includes aspirin, which, like high blood pressure, contributes to bleeding. Some surgeons caution patients against taking even a single aspirin within two weeks of undergoing their operation.

Before any surgery is performed, you should be aware of the limitations of the various aesthetic procedures. Face-lifts are not eternal. The effects may extend anywhere from two years to twenty years, depending on the elasticity of the skin, amount of sun exposure (too much sun accelerates aging of the skin), alcohol and cigarette consumption (excessive use tends to affect the facial skin adversely) and your own particular aging pattern.

"Some people look the same for years, then may change drastically," says Dr. J. Goin. "If you do a face-lift on someone who's at the beginning of an aging plateau that will last for maybe ten years, they'll look great and the effects of the operation will be enhanced. If you do the face-lift right at the end of the plateau and they go through the change, then people say the face-lift didn't seem to do very much for them."

A face-lift does not halt the aging process like some medical stopwatch. You continue to age, and so does your face, except that it continues to look younger than it would have without the surgery. The same holds true for eyelid surgery. Eventually, the lids sag or the bags return. Like face-lift patients, many blepharoplasty patients opt to have a second operation. Women who undergo any of the mammaplasty operations should realize that they may lose some of the normal sensation in the breast. In the case of breast reconstruction, feeling is not returned to the area, nor is the new breast an exact duplicate of the lost body part. It is similar in terms of size and shape, but it is not the same.

Plastic surgery involves cutting and manipulating living tissue. This means you cannot have the surgery without some temporary pain, bruising, bleeding and swelling. Scarring is inevitable, but usually the scars are well tucked and hidden. Recuperative time varies from one person and one procedure to another. Generally, people who have had eyelid surgery or a face-lift can be up and about almost immediately, but they may not want to resume normal public activities until the healing process is complete, simply because they don't want to be seen with discolored, swollen features.

Usually two weeks are needed for complete recuperation from eyelid surgery, though again, you can go back to work the day after the operation if you wish. A face-lift takes almost six months to heal fully, but most women find they are back to normal routines in two weeks and men in two to three weeks. (Men have thicker skin, which is less likely to bruise, but they also have a more difficult concealment problem.)

Perhaps most unsettling to many face-lift patients is the numbness they experience following surgery. They literally cannot feel their faces, cannot distinguish between where they end and the world begins. This experience can be disconcerting, especially when you lie down to sleep and can't feel the pillow beneath your cheek. About one week after surgery, feeling begins to return to the face, but it may take a month before you feel yourself completely back to normal.

Of the breast operations, augmentation is the easiest and requires the shortest recuperative time. Breast reduction may involve three to four hours in the operating room and several days' stay in the hospital. Reconstruction may require one or more different operations, depending on the extent of the mastectomy and the amount of reconstruction to be done. The process may extend over a period of several months.

Physical complications from aesthetic surgery are uncommon, but they do occur. For example, with the eyelid tuck, too much skin may be removed from the lower lid, causing the lid to pull away from the eye (a situation that may require a second operation). Or a person may temporarily or permanently lose vision in an eye because of excessive bleeding and subsequent pressure on the optic nerve (this, too, can be relieved, but the situation itself is very rare). Approximately 1 to 2 percent of people undergoing a face-lift will suffer from an injured nerve that might make their expression or smile uneven. Of these, says Dr. Hugo, 85 percent will recover on their own in six to nine months. Also uncommon but possible are wound infections from breast reduction surgery requiring additional treatment.

For some patients, suspicion from their spouse poses a problem. "Planning on having an affair?" "Looking for greener pastures?" may be questions asked aloud or silently by the husband or wife of a cosmetic-surgery patient. Other patients may face depression, even though they are pleased with their surgery. "Any operation is stressful," says Dr. M. Goin. "People should be advised that if their temperament is one that responds to pressure by 'being down,' then they should expect this after the surgery." The reaction, she explains, is completely unrelated to the results of the surgery. It is merely a response to the stress of having an operation.

If you are considering aesthetic surgery, you should be aware that, today, many such procedures can be performed outside the traditional hospital setting. In a ten-year study comparing the rate of significant complications of face-lift and breast augmentation operations done on an inpatient versus an outpatient basis, Donald R. Klein, M.D., of Dallas, Texas, found no significant difference between the operations performed in either setting among the approximately 1,600 subjects surveyed.

With the possible exceptions of body sculpting (the surgical removal of excess fat and skin from the abdomen, buttocks, upper arms or upper thighs), reduction mammaplasty and breast reconstruction, nearly all aesthetic procedures can be safely performed on an ambulatory basis in the hospital, in a properly equipped surgical center or in the office of a board-certified plastic surgeon, says Dr. Klein, president of the American Society for Aesthetic Plastic Surgery, Inc. Age is not a criterion for selecting inpatient over outpatient status. Instead, one must consider the patient's general, physical and psychological condition, his or her attitude toward being in a hospital, economic factors (inpatient care is notably more costly) and whether the individual has someone to care for him or her at home. You cannot expect to have surgery, then to hop in a cab and go fend for yourself at home. You are medicated and should not be alone.

"If you are interested in aesthetic surgery for yourself, you can ask your family doctor for guidance and recommendations. Or talk to a satisfied patient about his or her own experience," says Dr. Klein. "Any of these approaches is better than reading newspaper ads, looking in the Yellow Pages or just simply guessing."

14

NOTES FROM A
HEALTH SPA

*You bet appearance is important to me. I want to be the
best-looking woman I can be—at any age. I believe that what
you put into something—yourself included—is exactly what
you get out of it, and for me looking good gives an overall
good feeling.*

—a fifty-three-year-old Chicago woman

Middle-aged Americans have discovered the health spa. In increasing numbers, men and women in the fifties age group are enjoying the variety of facilities and activities provided by the nation's health resorts.

There are approximately 2,000 health spas in the United States. They range from resorts that offer mineral baths and massages to full-scale residential spas that promise a complete range of exercise programs and specially designed dietary regimens.

Health spas vary tremendously but can generally be divided into three broad categories: spartan and inexpensive; comfortable and moderately expensive; luxurious and very costly. The resorts attempt to attract the kinds of guests who will be most comfortable at their respective facility, so they provide fairly well-detailed literature on what to expect. The regimen at one, for example, might include a daily plunge into an icy stream, while, at another, the schedule will call for a swim in a heated pool. One spa might offer a diet of fruit and vegetable juices, while a second resort will feature gourmet meals of meat and fish. If you are interested in attending a spa, it is basically up to you to shop around and compare facilities to see that you get what you are looking for.

Only a few of the health spas in this country have full-time physicians on staff, although many have doctors or other medical professionals on standby. In any case, it is best to check with your own physician first before embarking on a rigorous health spa routine or on one that is simply very different from your normal life-style.

No one actually *needs* a health spa to be healthy. You can be fit and vigorous following a personal regimen of exercise and a balanced diet, and you can also find a range of physical activities available in your community. There are, for example, over 2,000 YMCA and over 450 YWCA centers or facilities in the United States. Most offer physical fitness programs. Private health clubs are popular, especially in urban areas and most park districts, and many community colleges offer health-oriented programs.

Still, health spas remain as that enticing something extra, and —guests say—the experience is worth pursuing. Here is a sampling of comments offered by middle-aged men and women chosen at random from the guest list of one of the country's oldest spas. This is the health resort as seen through their eyes:

• Martha, fifty-two, an East Coast mother and homemaker: "It's a good experience, a catharsis really. I've never been active before, and now I walk half an hour every day."

• John (Martha's husband), fifty-five, buyer for a large retail store and a man who readily owns up to the fact that he smokes and enjoys a drink regularly at lunch and after work: "The health spa showed me that I can change, that I can break habits like the five-o'clock martini. I'm sticking to the diet, which I never thought I could do. I only attend three exercise classes a day, though—none of the really hard stuff. People like me have to be careful. You can't just go leaping into a heavy program of activity."

• Anne, fifty, a California mother of three who teaches English as a Second Language: "When I said I was coming here, a few of my friends raised their eyebrows. But I decided that when you're my age it's time to do the things you've never done before. I'm really glad I came and didn't listen to my friends. Everyone should do this at least once. I would like to repeat it once a year if I could. I wish I could get my husband here. He needs something like this desperately, but he thinks it's just a beauty spa for women."

• Frances, fifty-four, an Oregon real estate dealer who's been to the spa four times (once with her husband) and plans to return again: "Every time I come, I learn something that I can carry over to my daily life. But more than that, it's my escape, a chance to relax and get away from it all."

• One divorced woman has been attending the spa for sixteen years and feels comfortable here because to her "it's a good place for a woman to come alone."

• A former high-school wrestling instructor thinks it's a great place for a man. "I work out in a gym and use weights," he explains. "But I have had no flexibility training. This shows you how much you have to learn."

• At dinner one evening at the spa, a gray-haired woman who had taken a week's vacation from her job says simply, "It does as much for the mind as for the body." Everyone at her table agrees.

Notes from Inside an American Spa: One Week at the Gate of Health

In the spring, as you drive along the southwestern coast of the country, you proceed into a little bit of heaven. The earth is green then, and barefoot children on bareback horses glide silently through the meadows. The landscape may be parched brown in the summer, but that is difficult to imagine now as the bus carrying you from the airport to your destination careens around sharp, verdant curves and hurries past dark, dipping canyons.

In the distance, mountains seem miragelike in the overhanging mist. The drive sets a mood. And what could be better than a ride through this paradise to arrive at the gates of what is said to be one of the oldest and largest health spas on the continent, a place not without its own sense of promise and bliss.

"The people who go to those places are just a bunch of fat ladies wrapped in purple togas being massaged all day." That was one prediction of what one could expect to find at the spa.

Someone else said, "How terrific. You won't do a thing but lay by the pool all day."

Others had other speculations of what it would be like: Being greeted at the gate with golden slippers or having the chance to lose ten pounds magically in one week were popular ideas. There were predictions of being bored by "the idle rich" and of being overwhelmed by movie stars and celebrities, who were sure to be there.

Mostly the health spa was envisioned as a kind of machine. You —the overweight, sagging guest—enter at one end and are processed through corridors where unknown things are done to your body. Finally you emerge at the other end, a new person, a slender person.

In the mind of the average American, *health spa* translates readily into only one image: *fat farm*. In this respect, the average American is—at least in the case of the Gate of Health spa (not the real name of the facility)—slightly out of date. There's been a transformation. That same interest in health that has converted at least a portion of our society from a sedentary to an active life-style has also turned the fat farm into a fitness resort.

The biggest surprise at the Gate of Health is the lack of emphasis on losing weight. It is part of the program, certainly, but it is not the entire program, and unrealistic weight losses are neither promised nor encouraged. In fact, guests are told that a two- or three-pound loss is an attainable goal and an excellent achievement. Running shoes, not slippers, are *de rigueur*, and dawdling poolside, it is hinted, is not the thing to do. Of the group who came to this resort at least one-third are fifty or older. The guest list is heterogeneous by sex, race, age and interests. Not a celebrity is to be found.

On Saturday afternoon, when the guests arrive, the Gate resort looks like a quiet, idle, even lazy place. The setting seems more conducive to a long rest than a week of physical activity. There are bright flower gardens, graceful palm trees, splendid cacti and lovely green lawns to enjoy. Tiled fountains and gazebos, swimming pools and adobe cottages are scattered across the spa's sixty acres, where guests retreat every evening to private quarters undisturbed by radio, television or telephone.

Suddenly, the 5:00 P.M. greeting hour arrives. And orientation begins.

Words like *rigorous* and *strenuous* intrude upon the scene. The friendly hills behind the spa are not simply to be admired, we are told; they are to be climbed. The uncultivated field leading to the foothills is to be hiked, preferably once a day. The innocent-looking building in the core area of the resort houses four gyms. The heated pool—the largest of four—is for volleyball, for swimming laps and for water-resistance exercises (muscle-toning exercises performed against the weight or resistance of water). The outdoor pavilions are not for picnics but for fresh-air exercise sessions when weather permits, and the sandy trail that looks like a path is really part of the spa's Parcours (a two-mile-long jogging/walking trail with twenty different exercise stations located along the route for a "total fitness" workout).

We are informed—and Sunday morning we learn for ourselves —that at the Gate of Health the day begins at 6:30 A.M. with a morning hike and continues until 5:00 P.M. If you follow the recommended regimen, you will select a minimum of *seven* classes each day, alternating the more rigorous with the less taxing.

Activity comes first. The pedicures, facials, herbal wraps (fine linen sheets steeped in waters imbued with the herb of the day, then wrapped around your body), saunas and massages are the rewards, not the mainstream. You are here not to be *put* into shape but to *get* into shape, and the distinction is vital. You will take from your stay only as much as you put into it. Your reward will be increased vitality, a pride in your accomplishments and, it is hoped, a carry-over to a healthier life-style after you depart.

The exercise classes at the resort last about forty-five minutes each and fall into one of four categories: aerobic—to stimulate cardiovascular activity and increase lung capacity; stretching— considered especially important for middle-aged people; relaxation—teaching the mind and body to let go of tension; and strength classes—to develop muscle stamina, either with weights or without. Guests are encouraged to try some of each for good balance. (People who lead a "rat race" type of life often select fast-paced exercises, such as running, and need to take time for slowing down, as in a yoga class or an afternoon walk.) The word at the spa is: Try to do something you've never done before.

In addition to these programs, there are classes recommended for men only—the Gate of Health is one of the few spas open to both men and women year-round—and classes recommended only for the very physically fit. To illustrate the pace and range of activity, here's a typical three-day schedule of one particular woman guest (see chart on page 206).

Three Days Inside a Health Resort

	Day One	Day Two	Day Three
6:30 a.m.		Mountain hike (3 miles)	
7:00 a.m.	Morning hike (2 miles)		Morning hike (2 miles)
8:00–9:00 a.m.	Breakfast	Wake up exercise (15 minutes) Breakfast	Breakfast
9:00 a.m.	Gate of Health exercise (strenuous)	Body awareness (posture, alignment)	Tennis clinic
10:00 a.m.	Spot reducing	Massage	Gate of Health exercise (strenuous)
11:00 a.m.	Dance class	Water resistance exercises	Facial
12:30–1:30 p.m.	Lunch	Lunch	Jump rope (10 minutes) Lunch
2:00 p.m.	Herbal wrap	Body contouring	Afternoon hike (2 miles)
3:00 p.m.	Stretch & relax	Parcours (beginner)	Advanced stretch
4:00 p.m.	Yoga	Yoga	Swim & sauna

The official week at the Gate of Health begins with a one-day "virtue" fast, basically a liquid diet totaling 550 calories divided into six snacks, one every 2½ hours. It is entirely voluntary; the staff entreats you not to do it if you have high blood pressure, if you are diabetic, to simply lose weight (you'll drop pounds, but mostly water weight, which comes back quickly) or if you plan on starting your stay with a vigorous class lineup. The warnings and explanations come as we sit the first evening in the dining room.

Facilities at the resort are arranged to avoid the overly crowded sensation that can result from too much centralization and also to encourage the guests to move about. To get from one place to another you have to walk—maybe the equivalent of a few hundred feet or a couple of city blocks. When the old iron bell rings at mealtime, it is a message to your feet to start moving—past the tennis courts, gyms and pools, past the recreation center, to the dining room. There, during the day, you can look out onto the canopied patios set on either side or onto the vineyard, which hails back to the days when the ranch was brand-new and the grape diet was in vogue.

At night the focus is on dinner—always delicious and inevitably meatless—and on the announcements of special events for the evening (a nutrition talk, a beauty-grooming session or a movie). On Saturday night the pros and cons of the virtue fast are debated. On Sunday night, some rumors are confirmed: someone who had been on the virtue fast fainted, someone else had a terrible headache. One person became dizzy, and another felt too weak to move. Inevitably you learn that the people who developed the problems ignored the warnings given the previous evening. Suddenly, the guests realize, this is all serious business. Lots of fun, sure. But a new feeling of respect settles in. From now on, the guests are going to listen and take heed. They'll shape up and they'll do it sensibly.

Throughout the guests' stay, much attention is paid to developing a new understanding of the body, the importance of an active life-style and the relationship of quality food as quality fuel.

During the first day or so, much of the talk centers on food. Compared with years past, the offering at the resort is a veritable feast, in recognition of the fact that not everyone is present to lose weight. The director estimates that as many as 50 percent of the guests are not interested in shedding extra pounds, because they haven't any to lose.

Those who wish to diet are not forgotten, however. They are urged to follow a carefully established basic food plan that offers approximately 1,000 calories per day: fruit and beverage at breakfast, a vegetable or fruit plate from the salad bar with cottage cheese at lunch—no frills—and a low-calorie dinner. If you are really serious about losing weight, you can request a special platter of cottage cheese and tomato wedges as a substitute for any regular lunch or dinner. Dieters are told no bread, no eggs in the morning, no tacos at noon and no "no-nos" (potato salad, deviled eggs) at dinner. All of those are for the nondieter.

If there is one complaint among the guests, it is that they tend to think and talk about food quite often during their stay. There is no doubt that for many guests the Gate diet represents a sharp departure from their normal intake. No salt is allowed, though a sodium-free substitute is offered. No sugar is available, but guests can use honey. There is no meat or alcohol, but there are a lot of fresh vegetables, cheese, fruit, herb teas, coffee and fish, which is served twice each week. An extra is tangy acidophilus milk, which is fresh milk fermented by special bacteria and reputed to assist one's intestinal flora in some positive fashion. The milk is used in the spa's salad dressing and is also available by the glassful at every meal.

By midweek, some guests drive into the local town for a glass of wine and a steak, but, for the most part, they adhere to the dietary program offered at the resort. It is a point of pride with many. Even those who said that the first thing they will eat on the way home is a hamburger admit that they like the routine and will probably start eating a bit more healthfully after they leave.

As spas go, the Gate of Health falls in the middle category, extreme neither in approach nor in cost. A week's stay at the spa helps dispel the basic reservation that, somehow, to take advantage of such a resort is overly indulgent. There are no guilt feelings expressed by guests and no apologies from anyone of any age group.

Taking care of oneself and feeling good about oneself are concepts that do not fall into the category of luxury anymore. The guests at the resort are not frivolous; they are serious about fitness, good health and vitality. They are preparing themselves to function better at their normal routines and priming their bodies and minds to be at their best.

It is strange how quickly we adapt. A few hours at the spa and you feel that the level of peace and tranquility there is the norm. Until you leave, however, you don't fully appreciate the difference between how you live and how you lived for that one week.

Suddenly you again encounter the daily realities. You breathe deeply and see and feel the pollution hanging overhead. You are hungry and find nothing but a proliferation of fast-food/fried-food convenience restaurants. You have an appointment and traffic backs up for half a mile on the only road into town. Maybe that important meeting was a flop, and the next three weekends are booked solid with niece and nephew graduations and weddings. A health resort like "the Gate" lets you escape—for a while at least.

The Health Spa Philosophy: How It Can Apply to Your Life

It is interesting that the power behind two of the most prestigious health spas in this country is a woman in her fifties. To Barbara Tarmina, fitness is a way of life. Besides overseeing her resort programs, she lectures frequently on the subject and has had extensive experience setting up fitness programs for nationally known organizations.

Movement, relaxation, nutrition and joy, she says, are the four primary ingredients of life. Each, she believes, is essential for a full, rewarding existence, and each is attainable only if we strive for it.

Why are some people able to attain their fitness goals, while others never seem to succeed?

Because of a basic sense of values. The people who succeed are those who get satisfaction from achievement, who set goals and carry them out. What we advocate here has to be done for the self, not for someone else.

I think that, overall, goals come first and the need for good health comes second. People now have to accept the fact that they will live to their mid-seventies. They will have one-third more life than their parents and one-third more of the opportunities. They can do one-third more of everything—if they are fit and healthy.

What about people who say they are too busy for exercise or for eating properly?

If you're doing so many things that you're busy all day, then you need the extra energy that comes from fitness if you want to keep equally active during that one-third extra of life. We truly believe here that most of the degenerative diseases are accelerated by negative eating and movement habits.

We recommend that everyone participate in an exercise program three times a day: morning, noon and evening, even if it is just for a few minutes. I walk and run for one hour every morning before I begin my day. Then I jump rope and do some stretching exercises for five minutes before lunch and again at the end of the day before preparing dinner.

Television has unfortunately made us into a society of takers. You take something to cure anything that ails you. My goal is to make us into a society of doers. And by doing, you take charge. You enhance your life.

What about those who say that exercise is not practical in their life?

Well, it's their life. If they want it that way, fine. We have to ask some very basic questions of ourselves today. For example, what is going to happen to us between the ages of fifty and seventy-five? Are those going to be twenty-five more healthy years of life, or will we be content to peak at age fifty?

Have you seen examples of people in mid-life who have turned themselves around in terms of fitness?

I've seen many who have been literally "born again." Something happens, and they've got it. It can happen at fifty, or at sixty. They wake up one day and say, "This is it. I've had it. I'm going to do everything differently." And they do.

First of all, you must begin with the urge, the idea, and then decide, "This is what I want!" Then go and get it. Expect to work for it. Of course there has to be a common-sense approach, step by step. But only you can take responsibility for yourself.

At last we are beginning to recognize the connection between health and achievement. People look about at the losers and the winners among their peers. They see that the people who are achievers are usually the people who are fit.

15

RESHAPING THE FUTURE: MID-LIFE CAREER CHANGE AND RETIREMENT

Every year I live, I am more convinced that the waste of life lies in the life we have not given, the powers we have not used, the selfish prudence that will risk nothing and which, shirking pain, misses happiness as well.

No one ever yet was the poorer in the long run for having once in a lifetime "let out all the length of all the reins."

—Anonymous

In northern Tennessee, a fifty-two-year-old homemaker stirs a cup of coffee and stares woefully out of the kitchen window. She thinks about her husband at work, about her two children away at school, and about how she will spend the rest of this day and the others that will follow. Although it is only midmorning, her work is already completed. Alone in the unusually quiet house, she asks, "What am I going to do with myself?"

Midway through a staff meeting on new procedures, a middle-aged Iowa banker stifles a yawn and doodles on the note pad lying on the table in front of him. "More bureaucratic paper shuffling," he thinks to himself. "I don't need this aggravation anymore. I wish I could pack it all in, but what else can I do?"

In western Oregon, a journeyman printer, forced into early retirement by company cutbacks, attends a special luncheon held in his honor. He smiles as he accepts an engraved plaque and listens to the accolades offered by his former co-workers. But his calm exterior belies the turmoil and panic he feels inside. "What am I going to do now?" he wonders.

Like hundreds of thousands of their middle-aged peers scattered across the country, these three individuals are struggling with a familiar problem: how to alter their life roles or traditional occupations when changes in personal, familial or societal values and circumstances indicate the need or present the opportunity for such a transformation.

Wished for or not, change affects all of us during the middle years. Some changes can be anticipated. If we are parents, for example, we know that our children will mature and leave home. If we are employed, we know that we will eventually face retirement. Even the majority of those who are self-employed or who operate their own successful businesses realize that their current status quo offers no guarantees.

Many other life changes may come without warning, and are often abrupt. We may be laid off or dismissed from a position that we held for years. We may be suddenly widowed or divorced and forced to develop new sources of income and activity. We may abruptly crave independence from former roles, or we may redefine our job and work goals in such a way that previous occupations no longer provide the necessary level of satisfaction.

We cannot avoid change, but we can decide whether to make our life changes work for the better or for the worse. In mid-life, when many changes seem to have an impact upon traditional roles, the crux of the matter is how each individual answers the familiar question, What am I going to do now?

What surprises many middle-aged people is the fact that they do have options. In this chapter we will attack another common misconception of the middle-aged, one that says they cannot reshape the future. Using input from career counselors and those who work in "life development" areas, and from the real-life success stories of middle-aged men and women who found new opportunity, often in difficult circumstances, we demonstrate that there are, in fact, many answers to the question, What can I do now?

We all need to use our time in ways that give us satisfaction. We may be paid for our efforts, or we may labor from a sense of duty, love or enjoyment. But what we do with our time, talent and energies is vitally important to our overall well-being.

Our self-image, status in society, income level, sense of personal worth and, to a great extent, our sense of identity are linked directly to our roles and occupations. But what we do can also have a crucial impact upon our physical and mental health.

Charles Lewis, M.D., chief of General Internal Medicine and Health Services Research at the University of California at Los Angeles, cites stress as a principal health-risk factor for people in their fifties. Excessive amounts or extended periods of stress can have both short-term and long-range negative effects on psychological and physical health.

Mid-life stress can have many causes, but it often results from dissatisfaction with one's work or role in life. People reach age fifty and wonder, "How did I get here?" or "Is this what I really want to do?" They often become depressed by what they perceive as a limited degree of freedom. They may fear taking a chance and failing and are often torn by the question of what they will do next.

The dilemma facing the middle-aged, says Dr. Lewis, is deciding how to proceed with the mental self-portrait they had begun constructing many years before. "Suddenly people begin thinking of all the things they wanted the picture to reflect and they wonder, 'Is it too late?' " Increasing numbers of middle-aged individuals are discovering that, within reasonable parameters, it is not too late.

A man may not catapult from bricklayer to airline pilot; a woman may not be transformed from lawyer to ballerina. The individual who is tone-deaf may not become a violin virtuoso; the solitary soul may not suddenly find fulfillment as a community organizer. But within the framework of each life exist unrealized possibilities and long-ignored talents that may be developed and pursued. These hidden potentials can be used to create new challenges and interests. They can make life more satisfying and can enrich the individual personality.

For people in the fifties age group, a realistic goal is self-renewal through the method of personal rediscovery. To rediscover oneself means to dust off the talents, skills, interests and abilities that have virtually been put on a shelf for years. Rediscovery is the recognition of personal resources that have been forgotten and ignored because one lacked time, money or opportunity, or because family or career responsibilities superseded. To renew oneself means to rekindle and utilize one's forgotten resources to add dimension, purpose and challenge to one's existence. When we are renewed, we escape boredom, dullness and contempt for the overly familiar; we channel our efforts into activities and roles that are exciting and fulfilling.

The Path to Rediscovery and Renewal in the Middle Years

Whether you are re-entering the job market after a long absence, contemplating a career switch or planning for retirement, the same basic three-step process of rediscovery and renewal applies to your situation. The first step is to identify your skills, talents and interests. The second step is to evaluate your resources and to clarify which remain important to you at this stage of life. The third step is to match your resources with the larger needs of society and of the marketplace.

"If you want to make a successful role change or enlarge on your range of activities, you have to start by looking at yourself in a different light," explains Nancy H. Navar, Re.D., a University of Illinois, Champaign, educator who has had extensive experience working with adults in a rehabilitative work-training program. "To a very large extent, our activities and roles are dictated by the view we have of ourselves. If we assume that our current activities reflect our only competency areas, then we cannot change what we do. But if we learn to think differently, then we open the door to acting differently. When we create a different mental picture of ourselves, we automatically provide new routes for behavior."

Alene H. Moris, director and co-founder of the Individual Development Center Inc., Seattle, Washington, one of the nation's first life-planning counseling centers for adults, has talked with thousands of middle-aged men and women who are faced with the prospect of mid-life career change. She has found that, often, the middle-aged are plagued more by negative attitudes than by lack of specific skills.

First, the middle-aged tend to focus their attentions on the credentials they lack rather than on those they have. If you do this, you can easily convince yourself that you have no options because you may not have earned a college degree or because you do not have an established track record in a given field.

Second, by mid-life, adults also have a tendency to think only in terms of the specialized roles they fill. This is natural considering the emphasis that society puts on specialization, but if you fall into this pattern, you can easily develop a very narrow view of yourself. You attach a label to yourself and then you let the label dictate your actions.

Thus, the aerospace engineer cannot see beyond his scientific training and skills. If you ask him what he does, he says, "I am an engineer." If you ask about his other talents, he says he has none, forgetting that he might do a beautiful job refinishing furniture or might also be an accomplished sailor. Similarly, the middle-aged homemaker claims that her only talent is in the kitchen. She forgets that as a fund raiser for a local mental health clinic, she brought in more money than anyone else ever had before.

"When we label ourselves, we tend to think we cannot do anything but what the label dictates. This is nonsense. We all have many talents. The challenge lies in rediscovering what they are," says Moris.

STEP ONE: IDENTIFY YOUR TALENTS

Before you can embark upon any mid-life change, you must know where your talents lie. You need a realistic picture of yourself. You need an accurate self-image that tells who you are and what you can do.

The information you require is at your fingertips; it is woven into your personal history. Your challenge is to recall and to make an inventory of the things that you have done, are capable of doing and that you enjoy. Here is how you can do this:

• *Review the most satisfying periods of your life.* If you want to change what you do and are seeking an occupation (paid or non-paid) or activities that will give you a high level of satisfaction, then you need to find out what gave you satisfaction in the past. When you look to the past, it does not mean that you intend to repeat what has already happened in your life. Rather, you are looking for clues, for bits and pieces of yourself, that, in the future, can be recombined or reshuffled into creative new patterns.

To complete this first step, identify the three most rewarding periods of your life, disregarding age guidelines and chronological sequence. After you have identified those periods, analyze them to determine what happened during those times to make them so rewarding.

First, list the three time periods. Then, next to each, write every task or experience with which you were involved. Note as many specific activities, responsibilities and interactions as you can remember.

This review technique was developed by Moris especially for people who do not have a history of formal employment and who feel intimidated by the standard approach to identifying job skills. However, even if you have worked throughout your adult life, you will benefit from this type of self-analysis. It gives you a different perspective from which to approach your life.

• *Review your life roles in chronological order.* This is a standard technique utilized in various forms by most career and life-development counselors. Although it follows the pattern of a formal employment résumé, it is also useful for people with a sporadic work history or none at all. The purpose of the technique is to develop a chronological review of your activities, pinpointing the specific skills utilized in each.

Beginning with your teenage or early adult years, list every job, avocation, volunteer activity or occupational role you have ever held or in which you have participated. Next to each one, write the specific skills you employed or the functions you performed, including those which, although not part of the official job description, were essential to your performance. For example, a former secretary might list not only typing, filing and phone answering, but also "ability to get along with people" and, if applicable, even tasks such as "proofreading" and "scheduling of meetings."

• *Review your "other" skills.* To complete an assessment of your competency areas, you must also consider the "other" skills. These are talents and abilities that might not be identified by either of the foregoing techniques. They are legitimate bits and pieces of yourself that provide additional clues to your likes, dislikes and competencies.

The following twelve skill-assessment questions are based on a competency profile developed by Dr. Navar and Carol Ann Peterson, Ed.D., also of the University of Illinois. Answer as many of the questions as you can. You can give more than one answer to each question, but you should not use the same skill or activity more than once. Sample answers are given in parentheses after each question.

1. What physical skill can you perform alone?_____
   (painting, animal grooming, automechanics, jogging)
2. Do you have a physical activity in which you can participate with others, regardless of your competency level?_____
   (walking, bird-watching, bowling)
3. What physical activity can you perform that requires the participation of one or more people?_____
   (tennis, fencing, dancing)
4. Do you have an outdoor activity or skill?_____
   (skiing, swimming, gardening, fishing)
5. Do you have a physical skill with carry-over opportunity in later years?_____
   (swimming, golf, walking)
6. What mental skill can you perform alone?_____
   (writing poetry, reading, crossword puzzles)
7. Do you have a mental skill you can perform with others regardless of your competency level?_____
   (playing cards, planning a social or charitable project)
8. What mental activity are you involved in that requires the participation of one or more people?_____
   (chess, book club)
9. What activities do you participate in as a spectator?_____
   (listening to music, watching a football game)
10. In what creative activities are you involved?_____
    (photography, woodcarving, playing the piano)
11. Do you have any skills that allow you to enjoy or improve your home environment?_____
    (cabinetmaking, cooking)
12. What are your community-service skills?_____
    (teaching first aid, chairing the church finance committee)

STEP TWO: CLARIFY VALUES

After you identify your skills and competency areas, you must evaluate them. Clarifying values simply means rating your resources on the basis of personal likes and dislikes.

The simplest way to evaluate your personal resources is to put a circle around every activity or skill on your lists that you enjoyed doing. Look for those activities and roles that were stimulating and rewarding. Focus on the activities that boosted your ego and your energy levels, the ones that gave you a real sense of satisfaction. Once you have done this, try to determine which specific aspects of an activity or role appealed to you. Why did you enjoy a particular position or period in your life? Was it the nature of the work or activity, the responsibilities you had or the human interaction involved? Almost inevitably, individual patterns will develop. These patterns, says Moris, provide additional insight into the type of person you are and the kinds of roles you might want to pursue.

For example, an accountant discovers that the aspect of his job he most enjoyed was working with people in financial distress. He also realizes that at another point in his life, while serving on his church board or community council, he played the role of peacemaker and again enjoyed the challenge of helping people who were in a stressful situation. "This man wants a change from accounting, but does not know what he should do," says Moris. "Perhaps he should consider a position as a labor negotiator? The job would utilize his knowledge of finances and numbers as well as his experience as a mediator, an experience he found very rewarding. For him, identifying and recombining specific skills and interests points the way to an optional career he might otherwise never even have thought of."

Values clarification also means putting activities and skills in perspective. On a separate sheet of paper, list your twenty favorite skills and activities chosen from among those circled. Next to each, note the last time you participated in or performed that activity or skill.

According to Dr. Navar, it is not unusual for people to discover large discrepancies between their perceived values and their daily activities. You may find that it has been ten or fifteen years since you last utilized a personal resource you claim is very important in your life. If this happens, the choice is then either to change your behavior and begin doing the things you say you enjoy, or to reconsider your values.

STEP THREE: MOLD YOUR SKILLS TO SOCIETY'S NEEDS
Finally, to effect successful change, you need to develop a sense of career awareness.

"Whether you are seeking a paying job or a volunteer activity or want to start your own business, you must study the environment and find out what needs to be done," says Moris. "It is very discouraging to prepare yourself to do a task that no one wants done. You only prepare yourself for disillusionment and disappointment. To succeed, you must fill a need."

What needs to be done? Moris suggests that you search for clues, both in the surrounding environment and within yourself.

First, look to newspapers, magazines, television shows, radio programs and conversations with friends. You have found a need when you feel your interest level rising or when you find yourself asking, "Why isn't someone doing something about that?"—be it the high cost of fresh produce, a lack of day-care facilities for young mothers, a local transportation snafu or the plight of widowers unskilled in home-care techniques.

Second, use your imagination. Pretend that you could ask a fairy godmother to grant you one wish to help improve your community or to make life a little more pleasant. For what would you ask? A better mousetrap, a good tailor, a used bookstore? When you answer the question, you have identified a possible need.

The next logical question to ask has to be this one: Why not me? Why can't I be the one to fill that particular need?

Coping with the Fear of Change

The prospect of change often prompts fear of the unknown and fear of failure. But sensible action lessens fears. Life review, skill identification, values clarification and career assessment are all sensible actions aimed at reducing the real fears mid-life change can present.

Too often, people want to change but are afraid that what they will do in the future will not measure up to past accomplishments, either in terms of status or income. This, however, should not be a hindrance to change. You are creating a new life for yourself— not reliving your past. Your new, second life should be judged on its own merits.

People may also hesitate to change because they perceive their future as being limited. This concern was more of a problem for previous generations. We have noted many times that society's view of the middle-aged has undergone a drastic, positive change. In addition, the natural extension of the life span nullifies the notion that at mid-life there is little useful time left. In fact, the average adult has many more years to enjoy.

Time and one's use of it is another problem. Throughout much of early adulthood and well into the middle years, familial and occupational responsibilities have largely dictated the expenditure of time. But, by middle age, the circumstances of our lives have altered, and many of our prior responsibilities have been greatly moderated. We can claim more time for ourselves. More than we may realize, we have the opportunity to do the things we want to do.

There is no doubt that change can be frightening, says Moris. "To make the leap, you need a new vision of yourself and of how you can be functioning in the world. The prospect can be frightening. But, on the other hand, the rewards are so fantastic."

To change, you need courage, she explains. You need the courage that comes from knowing yourself well and from believing in your personal right to a rewarding and fulfilling life.

True-Life Examples of Role Change during the Middle Years

The following are true-life examples of men and women who, during their fifties, either changed careers or roles or altered their life's activities in a rewarding fashion. Their personal experiences, skills and motivations vary tremendously. Yet each of these individuals achieved the common goal of self-renewal and did so through the process of personal rediscovery.

Faced with the question "What am I going to do now?," they forged their individual responses. Their experiences are a testimony to the hidden strengths and unrealized potentials of the middle-aged.

FROM VOLUNTEER TO PAID-WORKER STATUS

Carrie Dunset was nearly fifty years old when she began to feel vaguely restless and bored with her life. For her, these were new and disconcerting sensations.

For more than twenty-five years, Carrie, the wife of a skilled craftsman, had been a mother and homemaker. She had always found great contentment in fulfilling her obligations to her family, and she had never before questioned her role or her activities. But now, she realized, the circumstances of her life had changed. Her daughter, a recent college graduate, was completing a stint as a student teacher and would soon move into her own apartment. Her son was a high school senior and in a few months would be away at the local university. The truth was that Carrie's children simply did not need to rely on her as much as they had in previous years. "What now?" she thought.

For nearly one year, Carrie kept busy by decorating and arranging the new home she and her husband had recently purchased. Finally, when there were no more walls to paint and no more draperies to hang, she faced the reality of her existence. "There is nothing to do," she said to herself.

That morning, Carrie Dunset decided she needed more than her dwindling homemaking chores and her lifelong hobbies of reading and sewing to fill her life. "I knew I had to get out of the house and do something with myself," she explains. "But my prospects seemed awfully dim."

Because she felt unqualified for even the simplest paying job and because she still felt obligated to devote most of her energies to the care of her home, Carrie would consider only a part-time and volunteer activity. Because she did not drive a car and she lived in a suburban area that provided no public transportation, Carrie had to find an activity that was within walking distance of her home.

Even given these restrictions, however, Carrie Dunset discovered that she did have one option: a local school that served the mentally retarded and physically handicapped.

"I wasn't sure what they did at the school," she explains. "I had never had any contact with the handicapped, and I had no qualifications for working with children other than having been a mother for many years. I didn't even know if the school needed or wanted volunteers, but I decided, in the end, that I had to call. That was the only way I would find out."

When she finally dialed the number of the school, Carrie Dunset's heart was pounding. She secretly feared that whoever answered the phone would laugh at her offer to be a volunteer. "Instead," she says, "they were overjoyed."

Almost immediately, Carrie Dunset went to work. Once each week, she walked three blocks to the school and spent an entire day, from 9:00 A.M. to 3:00 P.M. assisting the teachers in charge of the younger students. Her chores were basic, but she found the interaction with the children to be highly rewarding.

Six months later, to her complete surprise, Carrie Dunset was asked to join the full-time staff as a paid teacher's aide. "I said *yes* immediately," she explains, "not because of the money, which was insignificant, but because, in that short time, my personal values had begun to change. I realized that so many of the things in my life that I had considered vital were really not that important. I did not need four days a week to wash windows and dust knickknacks. The school and the children had become more important than my busywork at home. This was clearly my choice, and I chose to become more involved with the school."

Carrie Dunset would have been happy to remain a teacher's aide. But she discovered, as so often happens, that one opportunity inevitably leads to another. Encouraged by her children and her husband, Carrie accepted each new challenge handed to her. As her expertise expanded, so did her self-confidence and her personal ambitions.

Today, at age fifty-nine, Carrie Dunset is manager of the school's adult workshop. She supervises an eight-member staff and sixty-two student workers, who complete simple assembly work on a contract basis for a host of outside clients. It is a well-paying, prestigious and challenging position.

"In my wildest dreams, I would never have imagined myself in this situation," she says. "But here I am, and I love it."

ALTERNATIVE WORK ARRANGEMENTS

For Carrie Dunset, as for thousands of other people in the fifties age group, volunteer activities opened the door to mid-life role change. For many other middle-aged people, however, the key to change may lie elsewhere. One possibility is the alternative work arrangement.

Twenty or even ten years ago, there was virtually no such thing as an alternative work arrangement. Today a number of unorthodox work styles are fairly commonplace in the work environment. Here is a look at some of the innovative arrangements that are changing the way people work.

• *Job sharing.* An arrangement in which two or more employees share responsibilities for one traditional position. Today many companies and civic agencies utilize job-sharing arrangements.

• *Temporary work.* A survey of 300 corporations reveals that 84 percent employ people on either a temporary or a part-time basis. Working mothers, students and retirees, in that order, constitute the bulk of this working population.

• *Permanent part-time.* The terms are self-explanatory; these are jobs designed to be part-time slots for extended periods. Today more than 20 percent of the labor force is employed in this fashion.

• *Flexitime.* Approximately 13 percent of all private firms with more than fifty employees offer flexitime, a system that allows workers, within limits, to set their own work hours.

Alternative work arrangements are a boon to the middle-aged worker. They are useful entry tools for persons returning to work and for those considering a career switch. They are becoming increasingly popular among both sexes as alternatives to traditional retirement arrangements. They also offer viable options to middle-aged workers who are either disenchanted with or, as in the following example, are forced out of the traditional labor market.

When Anthony Perko was fifty-two years old, he was pressured out of his job as an advertising and sales-promotion executive by internal policy changes in his company. In the ensuing months it became increasingly clear to Anthony that re-entry into his chosen field was not going to be an easy task. "Advertising is considered a young man's game," he explains. "I am sure my age worked against me."

While unsuccessful job interviews sapped Anthony's morale, child-support payments for three teenagers drained his savings. Finally, in desperation, Anthony joined an organization devoted to helping locate employment possibilities for middle-aged executives.

Although Anthony still hoped for an offer in advertising, none materialized. Instead, he was asked to assist the organization's public relations committee. He did, and through these efforts he established contacts that led eventually to two part-time jobs. One was as sales promoter for a midwestern industrial medical clinic and the other was as marketing surveyor for an eastern firm.

Four years later, Anthony Perko is still working—on a permanent part-time basis—in these two jobs. He considers himself 85 percent employed; he earns a "moderate living" (he is now paying child support for one son only); he also enjoys certain benefits denied to the traditional full-time job holder. "I have my own hours and more free time to pursue other interests," he explains. "I am also basically my own boss."

Successful part-time employment proved a financial and emotional godsend to Anthony Perko. It has also drastically altered his attitude toward future employment. "Before, I desperately wanted to get back into advertising," he says. "Now I would say there is a fair chance I will never return on a full-time basis to a regular advertising job. Through my part-time work, I have developed options, and this has made me much choosier about accepting full-time employment. I know I would never accept what I considered a mediocre job. I could not imagine giving up what I have for that."

USING EDUCATION TO GET AHEAD

Just as the middle-aged person can utilize alternative work arrangements to further his own options, he can also employ new, alternative educational opportunities to facilitate career and role change.

Today, there exists a wide variety of different ways for the middle-aged man or woman to make learning a lifelong venture. Equivalency tests, weekend college programs, summer courses and continuing- or adult-education programs are just some of the educational alternatives available. Public and private universities and colleges, community colleges, community centers, private corporations, church groups and national associations (such as the YMCA and the YWCA) are just a few of the institutions that provide access to new educational programs. In today's world, if you want to attend school, you will not be wanting for resources. No matter what your motivation or needs, the educational system can provide for the middle-aged adult.

And middle-aged adults are responding in record numbers to the opportunities. According to the latest figures available, approximately 18 million adults in this country are enrolled in credit and noncredit educational programs. Of that total, more than 10 percent are men and women aged fifty-five and over.

In New York, the fifty-five-year-old president of a prestigious film production company earned a long-coveted college degree through an external-degree program offered by the state university system. Although he had taken a smattering of college courses over the years, he was lacking sixty credits to qualify for a bachelor of arts degree. He earned three credits for passing a basic course in mathematics. He was awarded the remainder of the credits after an extensive oral examination, during which a group of professor-level evaluators quizzed him on his knowledge of film and media history and techniques. Although the diploma has no effect on his current work, it does much to boost the producer's morale. It will also make it easier for him someday to pursue his secret desire to teach history.

In another instance, a fifty-three-year-old West Coast widow enrolled in a training program at a center for displaced homemakers in the hope that the program would help her secure a job. The woman, who was in desperate financial straits, had no formal education beyond high school and had never worked outside the home. Her only identifiable asset was being able to speak both English and Spanish. The program counselors honed in on this talent. With their assistance, the woman learned to use her skill in community-service work. Eventually, her contacts and persistence were rewarded, and she landed a job helping coordinate a local bilingual assistance program for the elderly.

For a middle-aged retired North Carolina secretary, a degree in music provided both prestige and income-producing opportunities. For many years, the woman had sung in church choirs and played the piano for her own enjoyment. Still, she considered herself an untrained amateur. When she took early retirement, she planned to supplement her income and occupy her time giving piano lessons to neighborhood children. Before she could justify charging a fee for her expertise, however, she felt she needed formal training and a degree. Today, her diploma hangs on a wall in front of her piano, in full view of her young students and their parents.

DUSTING OFF HIDDEN TALENTS

Earlier we said that part of the rediscovery process is the full utilization of personal resources that previously had been slighted. At mid-life, rediscovery of hidden potential can result in important life-style changes that can revitalize and redirect the individual.

For Chester Watt of southwestern Colorado, for example, carpentry work had never been more than a necessary pastime. In retirement, it became an emotional lifesaver.

Chester was fifty-four years old when he left the postal department after twenty-three years of service. As a postal clerk, Chester had enjoyed his work. When he was promoted to supervisor, however, he began to chafe under the rein of bureaucratic procedures and restrictions imposed on him. Retirement represented his only way out of an unpleasant situation. Although Chester initially considered early retirement a blessing, only three weeks after accepting his gold watch, he began to have second thoughts about the wisdom of his decision.

"I didn't need additional money, but I did need something to do. I was incredibly bored," he explains. "I was sure that there was some function I could fill, so I began reading the want ads, looking for a job. When I saw an advertisement for a carpenter's helper—no experience needed—I called about an interview."

Chester's carpentry skills were self-taught and limited to home-repair jobs. In the previous three decades, he had completely finished the interior of his own home, built room additions when his two children were born, constructed utility sheds on his ten-acre plot and taken charge of minor repairwork for his mother, who lived nearby.

"Certainly I was apprehensive about the interview," he says, "but I thought that if someone else could do the job, so could I. For the interview I decided either to ignore or to emphasize my carpentry experience, depending on what the job required."

As it turned out, the opening was in the area of home construction. Chester was ideally suited for the position. His interviewer and potential boss, who was twenty years his junior, hired the retired postal worker on the spot. The next day Chester began working full-time at a job he had always enjoyed. Ironically, he says, he outperformed two younger men, ages nineteen and twenty-four, who had been hired at the same time.

For Chester Watt, mid-life role change resulted in his being formally employed by an established firm. More often, however, the process of change creates entrepreneurs who devote their talents to building their own businesses.

In Illinois, for example, a fifty-seven-year-old butcher sold the shop he had owned and operated for thirty years and began a new life as a wood-carver. Where once he whittled between customers in the back of his shop, the foreign-born entrepreneur currently plies his new trade in the garage of his suburban home. Now a full-time artist, he can hardly keep up with the demand for his work.

Similarly, in Connecticut, an independent insurance agent was able, at age fifty, to rekindle an interest and talent in pottery making. Although he revitalized his old hobby "just to have something to do," he soon discovered that people were more interested in buying his handcrafted pots than they were in purchasing insurance policies. Today, pottery is the man's job and insurance his sideline.

And in California, a fifty-three-year-old homemaker successfully turned a penchant for gourmet cooking into a lucrative career when she began giving French cooking classes in the family kitchen. Her business began quite accidentally when the woman showed a few friends how to use the then newly introduced food-processor kitchen appliance. For many years, the amateur gourmet had assumed that everyone knew his or her way around a kitchen as well as she did. When she realized she had an expertise, she took steps to capitalize on the talent.

According to Helen Hawkes, hidden talent is only one ingredient necessary for mid-life change. "On the basis of my own experience, I would say that to alter the basic structure of your life dramatically, you also need immense confidence and determination."

When Helen Hawkes was fifty-one years old, she traded in a twenty-year career as a high school English teacher for the uncertain life of a shopkeeper. The move was a gamble, but it was also the culmination of a dream.

For years, Helen had fantasized about owning her own business. When she traveled, she spent inordinate amounts of time investigating gift shops and talking to their proprietors. She developed a knack for spotting interesting and unusual houseware items. She also began a hobby of collecting antique furniture.

"The part of me that people saw was the structured, organized and conforming member of society. I was a teacher, wife and mother, and I worked hard at filling all those roles well," says Helen. "But the other invisible part of me was the dreamer, the adventurer, the curiosity seeker."

One day on her way home from work, Helen Hawkes noticed a FOR RENT sign in the window of a vacant neighborhood store. Suddenly, the pieces of her dream fell into place. Standing on the sidewalk, Helen saw her shop as she had long secretly envisioned it: gifts, antiques and natural foods on the shelves and herself behind the counter. "I was at an age when I knew I had to take a chance," she explains. "It was then or never."

Her husband was opposed to the idea, and her friends tried to discourage her, but Helen prevailed. "All I knew about business was that I had to buy a product and then sell it at a profit," she says. "I hounded house sales for inexpensive buys and I pleaded for credit from small suppliers. Initially, each step was a struggle and each tiny success a major victory."

Whenever the former teacher became discouraged, she threatened herself with the prospect of returning to her old job and the routine she had wanted to escape. She also thought of her mother. "She was a young immigrant widow with two children, left to run the family bakery in a northern Michigan mining country. If she could do it, without the education and other advantages I had, well, I thought, so could I."

Slowly but steadily, Helen Hawkes made a success of her business. She developed important contacts and attracted a growing following of faithful customers. Her husband, realizing how serious she was about the venture, capitulated and began offering moral support and helpful suggestions. Her friends stopped chortling and began questioning Helen about the basic rules of being an entrepreneur.

In a period of five years, Helen Hawkes expanded her shop three times. Eventually she was able to purchase the building that housed the store.

"The shop changed my life," she says. "I stopped wishing for things to happen and became more willing to take chances."

Her philosophy of life? "Do what your inner self tells you, and do it now."

DEVELOPING NEW EXPERTISE AT MID-LIFE

One popular myth about aging says that people are unable to acquire new work or leisure skills in mid-life or later. This is not true.

Advertising executive Anthony Perko, profiled earlier in this chapter, utilized part-time employment opportunities to learn two new and diverse job skills. Other middle-aged individuals are just as successful. By their experiences they demonstrate that even when one's options seem quite limited, opportunities can be developed. Following are two cases in point:

For all of his adult life, Edmund Niles had devoted himself to his wife, three children and his career as an educator. By the time he was fifty-eight years old, his children were happily settled on their own, his wife was involved with her own job, and he was kept more than busy as the director of elementary schools for a midsize Eastern school system. Edmund had every intention of working until he reached traditional retirement age when, suddenly, failing health forced him to relinquish his position. He was understandably despondent and spent most of his time rattling about in an empty house and brooding. Several months later, he suffered a major heart attack and underwent subsequent bypass surgery.

For nineteen long days, Edmund Niles lay in a hospital bed contemplating his future. He knew that he had to find some occupation to challenge and keep himself mentally stimulated. Reading, a lifelong hobby, would not suffice. But Edmund had no other skills or interests. All that came to mind was a vague, oft-repeated promise he had uttered through the years, a vow that, when he retired, he would take up the fine art of weaving.

"I had a choice of expending all my energy feeling sorry for myself or making good on my promise," he explains. "I decided there was more hope in the latter."

Edmund had acquired his initial interest in weaving from his mother-in-law. She had been a weaver for most of her adult life.

During the years she lived with Edmund and his family, he often watched her at work and marveled at the variety of practical items she was able to produce on the loom. In fact, her old loom still stood in his basement.

Once out of the hospital and back on his own, Edmund Niles enrolled in a local weaving class. (According to the American Craft Council, there are more than 2,000 places where instruction in various crafts are offered, both for the amateur and for the professional.) Edmund worried that the intricate mathematics involved in weaving might either stymie or bore him. He also worried that, because he was not "much of an artist at heart," he would not sustain an interest in the craft. However, after a few short weeks at the loom, Edmund Niles put his concerns to rest. He was hooked.

Today, Edmund Niles is a weaver. His handcrafted products include rag rugs, upholstery fabric and mohair clothing. Just recently, he turned down a request from the proprietor of a local store who was interested in selling his work. "That would have turned into a pressure situation," says Edmund, "and on doctor's orders, I avoid all pressure situations."

Edmund Niles estimates that he spends 50 percent of his time weaving (he now has three looms in operation simultaneously) and the rest on related activities. He is secretary of the local weaver's guild and proprietor of his own extensive library on the subject. Several times each year, he travels to weaving and craft conventions throughout the country. When at home, he regularly attends weaving workshops.

"I enjoy an immense satisfaction simply from having learned my skill," says Edmund Niles. "Each time I complete a project, this is reinforced. I can say with pride, 'I did that.' It's a marvelous feeling."

For Edmund Niles, being able to develop a new skill at mid-life meant a successful transition out of the hectic workaday world to which he was accustomed. For Liz Bondek, developing a new skill would mean the opposite. At mid-life, she needed a bridge that would facilitate her entry *into* the working world.

Liz Bondek and her husband did not part amicably when their thirty-two-year-long marriage ended in divorce. Liz was haunted by the thought that she had failed at the one venture most important to her in her life. She was also terrified by the prospect of having to construct a new life for herself. But she knew that she had no choice. No matter how much she analyzed her situation, Liz Bondek came to the same conclusion: She had to find a job.

She needed an occupation to fill her time. She needed more money than she had been granted in the settlement to continue living in a reasonable fashion. And she needed the satisfaction of proving she could be productive by society's standards. "How can you get a job?" her husband had said during the divorce proceedings. "You don't know how to do anything." To preserve her sense of self-esteem, Liz Bondek needed to prove him wrong.

"But what could I do?" she wondered. Before her marriage she had worked for a brief period in a candy store. She had no other formal work experience.

For weeks, Liz agonized over her situation. Step by step, she reviewed her life, searching for clues. "I realized finally that my years as a volunteer on the local school and community college boards had to be worth something," she says. "I began looking for the characteristics I had to have had to fill that slot. That is when I discovered my one strength—being able to work with people. I enjoyed and worked well with people. That is all I had to offer."

For many more weeks, Liz Bondek pored over the want ads in the local newspapers. Instinctively, she ignored the advertisements that emphasized a need for specific types of expertise. Instead, she looked for jobs that were people oriented.

"My first success was in a part-time position for a company that ran a small convention and meeting center. I greeted people, made up the daily list of events and answered phones. It was not very challenging and not well paying, but it was a start."

Several months later, Liz Bondek talked her way into a trainee position at a small travel agency. "I knew nothing about the travel business, but I knew how to accommodate people and I knew I could learn to do the job. Since I had traveled in the past, I also knew what irritated clients and what made them happy. I think the man who interviewed me was amused by my determination and my hard sell, but that was okay, because he hired me."

Although she was disappointed by the particular job she landed, Liz soon realized that the travel business could be the niche for which she was looking. During the next three years, she worked for several more agencies, using the experience garnered at one as her stepping-stone to the next. She learned the business, made contacts and enrolled in special training courses.

"I became an expert," she says. "I took the business seriously and poured every ounce of energy I had into making myself a success at it."

Twelve months ago, Liz Bondek cemented her new career. With two women partners, she became the owner and operator of an independent agency—one they claim is a little bit better and a little bit different from their competition.

"In this industry, it is almost unheard of to operate in the black in the first year. But we did it!" she explains.

There are times, says Liz Bondek, when she has trouble believing how successful and independent she has become. "I have survived what, in my mind, was the worst thing that could have happened in my life. I have made a success out of disaster. And I have created options for my own future. Now I will never be afraid of anything again."

REVITALIZING RUSTY JOB SKILLS

For many people, mid-life change can mean returning full circle to a skill or job enjoyed during an earlier period. When an Alaska dentist, for example, gave up a lucrative practice for the life of a commercial fisherman, he was going back to a world he knew well. As a boy, he had learned the trade from his father. Later he had put himself through college and dental school by working on large, commercial trawlers. When he turned fifty, he decided he had had enough of the everyday problems of managing a burgeoning clinical staff. He wanted a simpler life-style. The highly successful dentist, and father of four, did not have far to look for his second career. It was waiting for him at the water's edge.

For Mary Tunney, the route back through time was not as direct as the dentist's. The former nurse had to overcome what to her were seemingly insurmountable barriers posed by personal insecurities and out-of-date work skills.

"After I earned my bachelor's degree in nursing, I had worked for only one year, so I felt terribly inexperienced. And I also could not believe that, at age fifty, I would be an asset to any medical facility," she explains.

The first time someone suggested Mary return to nursing, she balked. "I thought the idea was ridiculous." Still, she admits, she could not tolerate the thought of being inactive once her seven children were grown. A few weeks later, when another friend urged her to enroll in a refresher course on nursing, Mary acquiesced. "But I took the course only because I had nothing else to do at the time.

"I refused to look for a job because I was stubborn and afraid. I thought, 'Who needs the humiliation of being rejected?' In the end, I suspect I was reluctant to consider the idea of nursing seriously because I was afraid of failing."

But Mary's friends persisted in their urgings. Finally she agreed to call about an interview for a part-time nursing position that was advertised in a local newspaper. "That morning, I said, 'Oh, they wouldn't hire me.' And that afternoon, they made me the job offer."

After thirty years of being a homemaker, Mary Tunney was again a nurse. She had been hired as a part-time laboratory instructor for freshman-level nursing students.

"I remember feeling terribly old and out-of-step," she says. "I felt I had missed too many years and could never catch up, and this caused many problems for me. I felt inadequate, and I did not like that feeling at all, because I had always been very competent and had always excelled at what I did. I missed having my former sense of confidence."

In her own mind, Mary Tunney had decided that she could not perform a job well unless she "knew everything there was to know about nursing." She admits that during her first year on the job, she was unhappy and disturbed by what she perceived as her own shortcomings. It seemed incongruous to her that, while she had such a low opinion of her own skills, her employer continually praised her performance. Finally, the offer of a second part-time position, coupled with the day-to-day experience of practicing and honing her skills, succeeded in allaying Mary's doubts and fears.

Mary Tunney is now fifty-eight years old. She works full-time as a nurse at a local hospital. She enjoys both her job and the sense of satisfaction that comes from knowing she is doing it well. Her self-confidence, she says, is at an all time high. Her sense of future is equally promising.

"After I realized I *could* be a good nurse, I decided I could be other things as well," says Mary Tunney. "And I began investigating other options."

Recently, Mary completed classes in sign language for the deaf. Today she is studying for a master's degree in adult education. On weekends she is a volunteer counselor for a local telephone crisis hotline.

"I am not unrealistic about what tomorrow will bring," she says. "But I am optimistic. I have discovered that our lives can be governed either by the attitude that says, 'No, I can't do that,' or 'Yes, I can.' I have opted for the latter. It has so much more to offer."

Many factors contribute to our overall sense of satisfaction with our lives. One ingredient that is very important is having a sense of choice over our own destinies. By the time we reach middle age, we may feel that we have relinquished or lost much of the art of being our own masters. In all likelihood, we have spent years subordinating ourselves to others: our children, our parents and our bosses. We may have found ourselves further restricted by financial and career responsibilities, by the unwritten sanctions of society that dictate attitude and behavior and by misconceptions and mythologies that emphasize only the negative aspects of human aging and thus distort reality.

This entire book is dedicated to the belief that, to often surprising extents, we have, at this age and time of our lives, choices we can make for the direction of our lives. The individuals profiled in this chapter succeeded in re-establishing domain over their occupational activities. Throughout these pages, we have seen other examples of people in their fifties who have triumphed over a variety of crises and misconceptions, discovering strengths and potentials they had never dared envision.

We have also talked with a myriad of people who are experts in areas of physiological and mental health. Without forsaking reality and acknowledging the very real problems with which people must deal, they are nonetheless optimistic about the rewards and joys that are possible in mid-life. With rare exceptions, these individuals are themselves either middle-aged or older. They speak from the experience of the scientific laboratory as well as from their own lives.

No one is guaranteed a happy life. No one is given easy answers to complicated problems. No one is spared a measure of harshness or injustice. For all of us, life changes. Some changes are positive, some are negative. But how effective we are in directing and responding to change—and thus in controlling our lives—depends on more than simply a roll of the dice.

"No matter how much of our life we perceive to be unchangeable, because it is in the control of someone or something else, there is always 'The Part' that we can work on to change," says Richard N. Bolles, director of the National Career Development Project, Walnut Creek, California. "Be it 2 percent, 5 percent, 30 percent or whatever, it is almost always *more* than we think."

Life-style, personal health habits and occupational roles are only a few of the factors that are within our direct sphere of influence. We can also choose to increase our knowledge, expand our range of activities and interests and modify personal attitudes and values. We cannot control the passage of time, but we can determine the stance we will take as our lives progress.

We can reshape our individual futures to fulfill the promise expressed in the words of the poet Robert Browning: "The best is yet to be."

SUMMARY: INGREDIENTS FOR GOOD HEALTH IN MID-LIFE

One of the most exciting and important findings of recent medical research is the discovery that middle-aged men and women can influence their health and overall well-being in positive and often dramatic ways. During the fifties decade you can take steps that will help you live better and longer.

Normal aging means *healthful* aging. Strange as it may seem, this concept is revolutionary. It is based on years of medical and scientific research, and it heralds good news for all of us. We can remain healthy and vigorous through the middle years, and indeed for the rest of our lives.

Equally startling is the documented evidence that links personal life-style to good health. Researchers have discovered that our daily habits and personal life-styles influence our physiological well-being far more than had ever been imagined. Heredity, of course, imposes its own limitations. Physiological resources vary from one individual to another. But we all share the ongoing opportunity to improve and to maintain our personal states of health. The methods are known. The challenge facing each of us is to decide to what extent we will utilize our personal physiological resources to ensure that we get the most out of our middle years.

We have a right to expect our lives to be highly satisfying during the middle years. But we must be willing to work for this goal. Good physiological functioning is a critical factor. By taking steps now to improve our physical health, we make an important investment that can yield rich rewards.

You can feel better, look better and be more active. You may become physically stronger and experience increased vitality. Good health helps us to enjoy an improved self-image and consequently to develop a more positive outlook. In short, we are preparing ourselves to live life to its fullest. In the long run, we may avoid premature old age.

Is it too late to start living healthfully now? Again, recent scientific studies provide more good news: It is never too late to adopt a sensible, healthful way of life. The sooner you begin, however, the more quickly you will start to reap the many benefits of improved health.

Here are the basic steps you need to take:

• Have regular medical checkups, as determined by your physician.

• Maintain a personal health profile that includes information about your medical history, previous surgeries and any medications that you take. Also include the medical histories of your parents and relatives.

• Be aware of changes in your behavior and physical functioning. Many of the behavioral and physiological changes that have traditionally been associated with aging may actually be symptoms of medical problems that can be treated and should be brought to the attention of your physician.

• Follow your doctor's prescribed treatment for any existing medical conditions.

• Take time for regular exercise and physical activity. It is always a good idea to check with your physician before you change your exercise habits in any way.

• Follow a sensible dietary program. Avoid the "fad" diets.

• Maintain a reasonable weight.

• Use alcohol only in moderate amounts.

• Eliminate, or use only moderately, cigarettes and other tobacco products.

• Learn how to cope with and therefore minimize stress.

• Take time just to relax.

• Learn to adapt to changes in your life. Flexibility is the key to coping with these changes.

Finally, take time for yourself. More than you may realize, you now have the opportunity to do many of the things that you have always wanted to do. Explore the many possibilities of your life, realizing that you hold the key to growth in your hands. You have earned your good health and vitality. If you use them to expand your horizons, you will enjoy an active, satisfying life both during your middle years and in the years thereafter.

NOTES

Introduction

xvi Dr. Bernice Neugarten's comments are included in a special report she delivered at the May 1978 annual meeting of the American Psychiatric Association in Atlanta, Georgia. The material was later published under the title "Time, Age, and the Life Cycle" in the *American Journal of Psychiatry* 136, no. 7 (July 1979).

xvii Sloan Wilson's personal comments about mid-life were published in the *Chicago Tribune*, April 25, 1981. They are included in an article entitled "Old Age: Where It's At, If You Can Get There" distributed by the Independent News Alliance of New York City.

xvii Dr. John Flanagan's data are taken from an ongoing, long-term study begun in 1960. The study is more fully discussed in Dr. Flanagan's "Quality of Life," which appears as a separate chapter in *Competence & Coping During Adulthood*, edited by Lynne A. Bond and James C. Rosen and published by the University Press of New England, Hanover, New Hampshire, 1980.

xviii Findings from the University of Michigan surveys of American attitudes are discussed by Professor of Psychology and Sociology Angus Campbell in a special interview article, "The Happiest Americans—Who They Are," published by *U.S. News & World Report* (December 24, 1979).

xviii   Data from the third study were gathered in a four-year analysis of life satisfaction among a cross section of adults aged forty-six to seventy. The subjects were drawn from the Adaptation Study at the Center for the Study of Aging and Human Development, Duke University Medical Center. The study was conducted by Erdman Palmore, Ph.D., and Vira Kivett, Ph.D. Their full report is entitled "Change in Life Satisfaction: A Longitudinal Study of Persons Aged 46–70." It was published in the *Journal of Gerontology* 32, no. 3 (1977).

xix   Dr. Paul Tournier's observations on aging appear in *Learn to Grow Old*, published by Harper & Row Publishers, New York, 1972.

xix–xx   Dr. Judith Bardwick's comments appear in an article entitled "Middle Age and a Sense of Future." The material was published in the *Merrill-Palmer Quarterly of Behavior and Development* 24, no. 2 (1978).

1 Good News about Health and Vitality in Mid-Life

10   On three different occasions, the Veterans Administration Cooperative Study Group on Antihypertensive Agents has published data from its long-term study on the effectiveness of antihypertensive drugs in reducing high blood pressure. The material cited here comes from an article entitled "Effects of Treatment on Morbidity in Hypertension. II. Results in Patients with Diastolic Blood Pressure Averaging 90 through 114 mm Hg," published in the *Journal of the American Medical Association* 213, no. 7 (August 17, 1970).

10   Initial findings from the nationwide National Institutes of Health hypertensive study are found in "Five Year Findings of the Hypertension Detection and Follow-up Program," published in the *Journal of the American Medical Association* 242, no. 23 (December 7, 1979). Further discussion of the data appears in "The 1980 Report of the Joint National Committee on Detection, Evaluation, and Treatment of High Blood Pressure," NIH Publication 82-1088 (December 1981).

11   The National Cancer Institute study was conducted by Sidney J. Cutler and Max H. Myers. It is reported in detail in an article entitled "Clinical Classification of Extent of Disease of Cancer of the Breast," published in the *Journal of the National Cancer Institute* 39, no. 2 (August 1967).

13–14   Dr. Lester Breslow's study of the health habits of nearly 7,000 adults began in 1965 and continued for 5½ years. A complete report is contained in an article entitled "Relationship of Physical Health Status and Health Practices" by Drs. Nedra Belloc and Lester Breslow. It is published in *Preventive Medicine* 1 (August 1972).

2 New Ways to Reduce Risks of Sickness and Disease

20 The Canadian health hazard appraisal study was conducted by Dr. John Milsum at the Division of Health Systems, University of British Columbia, Vancouver. The Arizona study was part of a four-year evaluation program headed by Sabina Dunton at the University of Arizona. The California survey was conducted by Dr. Joseph La Dou at the Ames Research Center of the National Aeronautics and Space Administration. All three projects are discussed in "Health Hazard Appraisal" by Lydia Ratcliff, published by the Public Affairs Committee, Inc., New York City. Pamphlet no. 558 (1978).

3 Coping with Everyday Physical Problems

27 The two-part University of Pennsylvania study compared sleep patterns of fifty smokers and fifty nonsmokers matched for age and sex and investigated the effect of sudden withdrawal from cigarettes on eight male smokers. In a report, "Cigarette Smoking Associated with Sleep Difficulty," a research team headed by Constantin R. Soldatos stated, "The results of these two studies suggest that cigarette smoking is associated with sleep difficulty." The article appeared in *Science* 207, no. 4,430 (February 1, 1980).

5 The Myths of the Mid-Life Crisis

40 The Bell Telephone employee study, officially called "The Management Process Study," began in 1956. It took investigators until 1960 to complete assessments of the original 422 participants. Eight years and twenty years after the study began, subjects were reassessed. Preliminary findings and the study itself are discussed more fully by Douglas W. Bray and Ann Howard in a report entitled "Career Success and Life Satisfactions of Middle-Aged Managers." The material appears as a separate chapter in *Competence & Coping During Adulthood*, edited by Lynne A. Bond and James C. Rosen and published by the University Press of New England, Hanover, New Hampshire, 1980.

40 Grace K. Baruch, Ph.D., and Rosalind C. Barnett, Ph.D., began their study of middle-aged women in March 1978 and completed research in March 1981. Preliminary findings are reported in "A New Start for Women at Mid-life," written with Caryl Rivers and published in the *New York Times Magazine* (December 7, 1980).

41 The Colchester Study of Aging surveyed attitudes of 600 men, women and children between the ages of five and eighty. The study, headed by John Nicholson, was conducted in Colchester, England. "Three Seasons of Life," a three-part series, reports the findings in *New Society* 53, nos. 926–928 (August 14, August 21 and August 28, 1980).

6 Easing the Stresses and Strains of Mid-Life

48 Meg Greenfield's comments appear in an article entitled "On Facing Fifty," published in *Newsweek* (November 5, 1979).

50 Elliott Jacques discusses the issue of personal mortality in an article entitled "Death and the Mid-life Crisis," published in the *International Journal of Psychoanalysis* 46 (1965).

53 The National Institutes of Health analysis of coping mechanisms was conducted by Leonard I. Pearlin, Ph.D., and Carmi Schooler. It is reported fully in their article "The Structure of Coping," *Journal of Health and Social Behavior* 19 (1978).

53 The Chicago coping study was conducted in 1972. It is discussed fully in the article by Frederic W. Ilfeld, Jr., entitled "Coping Styles of Chicago Adults: Description," *Journal of Human Stress* (June 1980).

59 The cognitive-therapy study was conducted at the University of Pennsylvania. It is reported in an article entitled "Comparative Efficacy of Cognitive Therapy and Imipramine in the Treatment of Depressed Patients," published in *Cognitive Therapy and Research* 1 (1977).

7 Understanding the Female Menopause and the Male Climacteric

63 The Tucson meeting, held in 1979, was the third annual gathering of the Society for Menstrual Cycle Research. Attending were researchers from the United States, Canada and Europe.

67 The first two reports that linked estrogen therapy to cancer were published in 1975 in the *New England Journal of Medicine*. The first was "Association of Exogenous Estrogen and Endometrial Carcinoma," by Donald C. Smith, M.D., Ross Prentice, Ph.D., Donovan J. Thompson, Ph.D., and Walter L. Herrman, M.D. The second was "Increased Risk of Endometrial Carcinoma among Users of Conjugated Estrogens," by Harry K. Ziel, M.D., and William D. Finkle, Ph.D. Both articles appear in 293, no. 23 (December 4, 1975).

67 The Baltimore study, which began in 1974, was conducted by ten medical researchers from four different medical institutions. Their report is entitled "Endometrial Cancer and Estrogen Use." It appears in the *New England Journal of Medicine*, 300, no. 1 (January 4, 1979).

67 The Boston Collaborative Drug Surveillance Program study utilized information on estrogen use taken from the records of the Group Health Cooperative of Puget Sound, Seattle, Washington, for a two-year period from July 1975 through June 1977. A complete report, entitled "Replacement Estrogens and Endometrial Cancer," appears in the *New England Journal of Medicine* 300, no. 5 (February 1, 1979).

67 Recommendations of the American Council on Science and Health appear in the council's brochure entitled "Postmenopausal Estrogen Therapy" (November 1979).

67 The National Institutes of Health Conference on Estrogen Use and Postmenopausal Women was held September 13–14, 1979. A summary of the proceedings is contained in a booklet entitled "Consensus: Estrogen Use and Postmenopausal Women," 2, no. 8. The proceedings also are reported in the *Annals of Internal Medicine* 91, no. 6 (December 1979).

68 Dr. Edward Tilt's comments originally appeared in his book *The Change of Life in Health and Disease*, published by John Churchill, London, 1857. They are reprinted in "Psychiatric Disorders Associated with the Menopause," Chapter 4 of *The Menopause*, edited by Robert J. Beard, M.T.P. Press, Lancaster, England, 1976, and University Park Press, Baltimore, 1976.

68 The negative portrait of the menopausal and postmenopausal women as drawn by Freud, Deutsch and others is explored in a number of works by contemporary researchers and writers. See, for example, "Menopause," by Connie Bruck in *Human Behavior*, April 1979; and *Menopause: A Positive Approach*, by Rosetta Reitz (New York: Penguin Books, 1977).

69 In their study of menopausal symptoms, Dr. Bernice Neugarten and Ruth J. Kraines, Ph.D., questioned 460 women, ages thirteen to sixty-four. Their findings are fully reported in an article entitled "Menopausal Symptoms in Women of Various Ages," published in *Psychosomatic Medicine* 27, no. 3 (1965). For the attitudinal survey headed by Dr. Neugarten, 267 women, ages twenty-one to sixty-five, were questioned. A full report,

"Women's Attitudes Toward the Menopause" is published in *Vita humana*, 6 (1963).

69   Dr. Ann Voda's study of hot flashes in menopausal women is now in its second stage. Her initial findings are presented in an article entitled "Climacteric Hot Flash," *Mauritas* 3 (1981), and in an article entitled "Menopausal Hot Flash" in *Changing Perspectives on Menopause* (Austin: University of Texas Press, 1982).

70   A summary of the hot-flash research conducted at the University of California, San Diego, is found in "Hot Flashes: More Than One Culprit," *Science News* (September 8, 1979). A full report of the findings is included in an article entitled "Menopausal Flushes: A Neuroendocrine Link with Pulsatile Luteinizing Hormone Secretion," *Science* 205, no. 24 (August 1979).

71   Subjects in the Duke University study are participants in an ongoing longitudinal adaptation study at the university's Center for Aging and Human Development. In this project, headed by Eric Pfeiffer, M.D., data from 261 men and 241 women, ages forty-five to sixty-nine, are analyzed. Findings are reported in an article entitled "Sexual Behavior in Middle Life," published in the *American Journal of Psychiatry* 128, no. 10 (April 1972).

71   A detailed discussion of the 1974 survey conducted by the Boston Women's Collective is found in "Menopause," Chapter 17 of *Our Bodies, Ourselves*, published by Simon and Schuster, New York, 1976.

75   Jacqueline Gretzinger and Kristi Dege completed their study in 1979. They report their survey findings on how menopause affects men in an article entitled "Attitudes Toward Menopause of Women, Their Husbands, and Their Children," presented at the annual meeting of the American Anthropological Association, November 1979. Data are also reported in "Attitudes of Families Toward Menopause," in *Changing Perspectives Toward Menopause* (Austin: University of Texas Press, 1982).

88–90   A full report of Dr. Richard Spark's study of impotence, conducted with Robert A. White and Peter B. Connolly, M. S., is found in an article entitled "Impotence Is Not Always Psychogenic." It appears in the *Journal of the American Medical Association* 243, no. 8 (February 22–29, 1980).

8 The Middle-Aged Person and the Family

95 The San Francisco survey was conducted by Lillian B. Rubin, Ph.D. Subjects ranged in age from thirty-five to fifty-four, and all were either married or once-married. Dr. Rubin's findings are discussed fully in *Women of a Certain Age* (New York: Harper & Row Publishers, 1979).

95 In the Colorado State University study, conducted by Clifton E. Barber, Ph.D., twenty-five men and twenty-five women, representing fifty families, were interviewed. Findings are included in a report entitled "Gender Differences in Experiencing the Transition to the Empty Nest: Reports of Middle-Aged Women and Men," which was presented at the 1978 meeting of the Gerontological Society of America.

96 The third research project, conducted by Linda Brookover Bourque, Ph.D., and Kurt W. Bach, Ph.D., utilized data collected as part of an ongoing longitudinal adaptation study at the Center for Aging and Human Development at Duke University. Some 371 subjects were interviewed over a four-year period. Data are fully reported in "Life Graphs and Life Events," *Journal of Gerontology* 32, no. 6.

102 The two-year University of Oklahoma study was completed in 1976. It is discussed in an article entitled "Strengthening Marriage in the Middle Years," by Maggie P. Hayes, Ed. D., *Family Perspective* (Winter 1979).

103 In the University of California, San Francisco, study, conducted by Majda Thurnher, some fifty-four middle-aged men and women were interviewed about their marital relationships. Findings are discussed in an article entitled "Midlife Marriage: Sex Differences in Evaluation and Perspectives," presented at the 1974 meeting of the Gerontological Society of America.

111 Lucy Bartel, Ph.D., spent one year studying the adjustment problems of sixty men and eighty-five women who had remarried after divorce. Her findings are reported in the dissertation entitled "Remarriage: A Study of the Factors Leading to Success or Failure in Remarriage," Florida State University, Tallahassee (1977).

9 Facing the Special Problems of Widowhood and Widowerhood

118 Data for the Scripps Foundation study were obtained in a survey of 1,106 adults aged fifty or older who lived in a rural

Midwestern township. Of the subjects, 161 were widowed. The study was conducted by Suzanne Kunkel and findings are included in a report entitled "Sex Differences in Adjustment to Widowhood," presented at the thirty-second annual meeting of the Gerontological Society of America in November 1979.

118 The State University of New York study is entitled "Widowhood and Well-Being." It was conducted by Diana Antos Arens, Ph.D., and was also presented at the meeting of the Gerontological Society of America in November 1979.

118 The St. Louis study, conducted by Aaron Rosen, Ph.D., and Arthur Shulman, Ph.D., began in 1977. It included a general survey of 850 widowed women and a detailed study of the coping strategies of 150 widows. Preliminary findings are included in several papers presented at the 1981 and 1982 meetings of the Gerontological Society of America. Final analysis of the data will be published in book form by the mid-1980s.

121 A report on the Yale University study, conducted by Selby Jacobs, M.D., and Adrian Ostfeld, M.D., is included in an article entitled "Fatal Widow's Weeds," in *Human Behavior* (October 1978).

121 Knud Helsing's nonconcurrent prospective study began in 1963 and ended in 1975. All subjects lived in Washington County, Maryland. Final data were reported in "Factors Associated with Mortality After Widowhood," *American Journal of Public Health* 71, no. 8 (August 1981), and in "Mortality After Bereavement," *American Journal of Epidemiology* 114, no. 1 (1981).

122 Jacqueline Lee Zimmer, Ph.D., compared sixty-one recent and long-widowed women over age fifty-five in the study at the California School of Professional Psychology. Her findings are reported in the dissertation entitled "Adjustment of Older Women to Widowhood," California School of Professional Psychology, San Diego, 1975.

122 In the Wichita State University study, Carol J. Barnett, Ph.D., studied the effects of group-therapy sessions among seventy widowed women, ages thirty-two to seventy-four. Her findings are discussed fully in "Effectiveness of Widows' Groups in Facilitating Change," *Journal of Consulting and Clinical Psychology* 46, no. 1 (1978).

123 The Detroit study was conducted by Amanda A. Beck, Ph.D., and Barbara Leviton, M.A. Persons in 2,500 households were

questioned about life satisfaction; 37 percent of the subjects were widowed. Findings are included in a report entitled "Social Support Mediating Factors in Widowhood and Life Satisfaction Among the Elderly," presented at the 1976 meeting of the Gerontological Society of America.

10 Sexual Functioning at Mid-Life

133 The clinical observations of William H. Masters, M.D., and Virginia E. Johnson, Sc.D., are found in *Human Sexual Response*, published by Little, Brown and Company, Boston, 1966. Their book includes special chapters on sexual functions in aging men and women.

136 F. Brantley Scott, M.D., directed the implant program at Baylor College. A full report by his research team is found in an article entitled "Erectile Impotence Treated with an Implantable, Inflatable Prosthesis," *Journal of the American Medical Association* 241, no. 24 (June 15, 1979).

138 The University of Pittsburgh study was conducted by Ellen Frank, M.S., Carol Anderson, M.S.W., and Debra Rubinstein, M.S. It is fully reported in an article entitled "Frequency of Sexual Dysfunction in 'Normal' Couples," published in the *New England Journal of Medicine* 299, no. 3 (July 20, 1978).

140 Comments are from the University of Pittsburgh study of 100 married couples mentioned earlier in this chapter.

11 Exercise and Sports in Mid-Life

149 Gallup poll survey data are discussed in an article entitled "The Fitness Mania," *U.S. News & World Report* (February 27, 1978).

149 Data from the President's Council on Physical Fitness and Sports are found in "An Introduction to Physical Fitness," DHEW Publication no. (OS) 79-50068.

151 National Institutes of Health comments are included in findings presented at a 1977, three-day conference on the role of exercise in preventing physical decline. The conference was cosponsored with the President's Council on Physical Fitness and Sports. More information is included in "Special Report on Aging: 1978," DHEW Publication no. (NIH) 78-1538.

151–154 In "Exercise as Protection Against Heart Attack," Ralph S. Paffenbarger, Jr., M.D., and Robert T. Hyde, M.A., review research findings of more than half a dozen recent study projects that credit exercise with having positive effects on the cardiovascular system. Their article appears in the *New England Journal of Medicine* 302, no. 18 (May 1, 1980).

152   The Duke University study is reported in an article entitled "Physical Conditioning Augments the Fibrinlytic Response to Venous Occlusion in Healthy Adults," *New England Journal of Medicine* 302, no. 18 (May 1, 1980).

154   The Swedish study of sixteen subjects was conducted over a thirteen-year period by Inge-Lis Kanstrup and Bjorn Ekblom. Their findings are reported in an article entitled "Influence of Age and Physical Activity on Central Hemodynamics and Lung Function in Active Adults," *Journal of Applied Physiology* 45, no. 5 (November 1978).

157   The studies at the University of Wisconsin, University of Illinois and University of Pittsburgh are among numerous research projects that link exercise to better mental health. For further reading, see "When You Don't Know What Ails You," by Lawrence Galton, *Parade*, December 9, 1979; *The Sportsmedicine Book*, by Gabe Mirkin, M.D., and Marshall Hoffman (Boston: Little, Brown & Company, 1978), and *The Exerciser's Handbook*, by Charles Kuntzleman, Ed.D. (New York: David McKay Company, Inc., 1978).

163   The exercise guidelines from the American College of Sports Medicine were first issued in 1978. They are discussed fully in an article entitled "The Recommended Quantity and Quality of Exercise for Developing and Maintaining Fitness in Healthy Adults," *Medicine and Science in Sports* 10, no. 3 (1978).

165–167   Every day, newspapers, magazines and local radio and television stations throughout the country report the feats of America's middle-aged athletes, such as the men and women featured in our Hall of Fame for Fifties. Our information sources include the following: *Sports Illustrated*, "Faces in the Crowd" Section (January 12, 1979; March 9, 1981; April 6, 1981; and June 16, 1980); *Chicago Sun Times* (September 15, 1979; and August 4, 1980); *Dynamic Years* (May–June 1981); *The Carsman* (January 1981); the publicity office of the Indianapolis 500 in Indianapolis, Indiana; and the National Standard Race Information Office (World-Wide Ski Corporation) in Aspen, Colorado.

12 Guidelines for Healthy Nutrition and Weight Loss

168 The article giving the overview of what is known about foods and nutrition as of 1981 appears in the *Journal of the American Medical Association* (June 5, 1981).

176, 177 Findings from two studies conducted under the auspices of the National Institute on Aging are reviewed in "Special Report on Aging, 1981," published by the U.S. Department of Health and Human Services, Public Health Service, National Institutes of Health, National Institute of Aging, NIH publication 81-2328 (September 1981). The studies are entitled "Taste Perception Study" and the "Study on Caloric Restrictions in Animals." The "Taste Perception Study" was referred to in the *Journal of the American Medical Association* (February 12, 1982) in the section "From the NIH," p. 775.

178 The guidelines for calorie reduction suggested by the National Academy of Sciences and the World Health Organization appear in the article "Recommended Dietary Allowances for the Elderly," by A. E. Harper, Ph.D., published in *Geriatrics* (May 1978).

13 Making a Decision About Cosmetic Surgery

191 Drs. John and Marcia Goin's full report on mastectomy/breast reconstruction patients is found in an article entitled "Mastectomy and Subsequent Breast Reconstruction in Midlife." It appears in the *Archives of General Psychiatry*, 38 (February 1981).

200 "A Comparison of Complications Between Inpatients and Outpatients for Aesthetic Surgical Procedures: A Ten-Year Study," by Donald Klein, M.D., and Allan Rosenberg, Ph.D., was presented at the annual meeting of the American Society for Aesthetic Plastic Surgery in May 1980. The findings were also published in *Plastic and Reconstructive Surgery* (January 1981).

15 Reshaping the Future: Mid-Life Career Change and Retirement

235 Richard Bolles' comments are found in *What Color Is Your Parachute?*, published by Ten Speed Press, Berkeley, 1981.

235 "Grow old along with me! The best is yet to be, The last of life, for which the first was made." The lines are taken from "Rabbi Ben Ezra," by Robert Browning, written in 1864.

Your Personal Health History

Below is a convenient chart for keeping track of your own medical history—information which will be helpful to you and your physician. The shaded areas are samples for you to follow in filling out the chart. Be sure to keep your health history data up to date and let a friend or relative know where you keep the information.

Medical Problems and Allergies

	Date	Nature of Illness	Physician	Comments (status of illness)
SAMPLE	11/1/80	High blood pressure	Dr. Smith	Daily medication required

Hospitalizations and Surgery

	Date	Hospital	Reason	Description (type of surgery)
SAMPLE	1/7/82	Northwest Memorial- Los Angeles	Heart pains	Bypass surgery

Medications You Take

Date	Name	Dose	Frequency
SAMPLE 1/5/80	Hydrochlorothiazide	5 mg.	One pill once a day in the morning.

Diseases of Your Blood Relations

Name	Serious Illness	Age at Death	Cause of Death
Mother			
Father			
Grandparents			
Brothers/Sisters			
Other			

INDEX

part-time, 92, 106, 223–24
retirement from, 41, 52, 92, 93,
　211–12
stress and, 213
temporary, 223
volunteer, 97, 221–22

see also career changes; career
　choices
Wynder, Ernest L., 11

Zussman, Leon, 141–45
Zussman, Shirley, 141–45

ABOUT THE AUTHOR

PATRICIA SKALKA, a free-lance writer living in Chicago, has written extensively for the consumer public. She is a former assistant managing editor of *Today's Health Magazine* and has written three previous books. Ms. Skalka was born in Chicago, Illinois, and received her B.A. in communications from the University of Dayton (Ohio).